Glucose Revolution:

Reclaim Your Health with Balanced Blood Sugar

By

Carlos P. Branch

Disclaimer

The content in this book is provided solely for educational and informational reasons and is not intended to be medical advice. Before changing your diet, exercise routine, or medication regimen, always talk with a trained healthcare expert. The author and publisher accept no responsibility for any negative effects or repercussions stemming from the use of any suggestions, preparations, or methods contained in this book. Individual results may vary, and the information in this book may not be applicable to everyone. The reader accepts full responsibility for any decisions or actions based on the information provided herein.

Table of contents

Introduction

Welcome to the Glucose Revolution!

Welcome to the "Glucose Revolution: Reclaim Your Health with Balanced Blood Sugar." This book is a complete guide to learning and mastering the complexities of blood sugar regulation, with the goal of transforming your health and wellbeing. As we embark on this adventure together, you will understand how blood sugar affects practically every part of your life, from energy levels and mood to long-term health and vitality.

Our bodies' major source of energy is blood sugar, sometimes known as glucose. It fuels our cells, powers our minds, and maintains vital physiological functions. When blood sugar levels become unbalanced, it can cause a slew of health problems, ranging from weariness and weight gain to more serious disorders like diabetes and heart disease.

The "Glucose Revolution" is about regaining control of your health by recognizing the critical role of blood sugar and implementing measures to keep it balanced. Whether you want to increase your energy, enhance your mood, lose weight, or prevent chronic diseases, this book will give you the information and techniques you need.

In this introduction, we will discuss the significance of balanced blood sugar levels, detail how to use this book successfully, and lay the groundwork for a transforming path to greater health.

Importance of Balanced Blood Sugar

A balanced blood sugar level is essential for overall health and well-being. When glucose levels are consistent, your body runs smoothly, and you feel energized, focused, and resilient. In contrast, blood sugar imbalances can cause a variety of short- and long-term health issues.

Short-Term Effects

In the short run, blood sugar abnormalities can induce symptoms like:

Fatigue: When your blood sugar levels soar and then drop, you may feel extremely weary and lethargic. This high-low cycle can make it challenging to maintain constant energy levels throughout the day.

Mood Swings: Changing blood sugar levels can alter your mood, causing impatience, anxiety, and even depression. These shifts in mood can have an influence on your relationships and overall quality of life.

Hunger and Cravings: Unstable blood sugar levels can cause severe hunger and cravings, especially for sugary or high-carbohydrate foods. This can lead to overeating and poor food choices, worsening blood sugar abnormalities.

Long-Term Effects

Chronic blood sugar abnormalities can lead to major health issues, such as:

Type 2 Diabetes: Persistently elevated blood sugar levels can cause insulin resistance, which is a major factor in the development of type 2 diabetes. This disorder affects millions of people worldwide and can lead to a variety of issues, including nerve damage, kidney disease, and visual problems.

Cardiovascular Disease: Elevated blood sugar levels can harm blood vessels, increasing the risk of heart disease and stroke. Maintaining stable blood sugar levels is critical for cardiovascular health.

Weight Gain and Obesity: Insulin resistance and high blood sugar levels can encourage fat storage, especially in the abdomen. This can cause weight gain and raise the risk of obesity-related health problems.

Cognitive Decline: New research reveals that blood sugar abnormalities may cause cognitive decline and raise the chance of acquiring neurodegenerative disorders such as Alzheimer's.

Understanding and managing your blood sugar levels is critical for avoiding serious health issues and maintaining good health. You may maintain balanced blood sugar and improve your quality of life by making informed decisions about your nutrition, lifestyle, and overall health.

How to Use This Book:

"Glucose Revolution: Reclaim Your Health with Balanced Blood Sugar" is intended to be a practical and comprehensive resource for anyone wishing to enhance their health by managing blood sugar more effectively. Whether you're a beginner or have some experience, this book will walk you through the process of understanding and achieving balanced blood sugar levels.

Structure of the book

The book is divided into several important sections, each concentrating on a distinct component of blood sugar regulation.

1. Understanding Glucose and Blood Sugar: This section provides an overview of glucose, how it works in the body, and the mechanisms that control blood sugar levels.

2. The Science of Blood Sugar: Here, we look at the molecular and physiological processes that influence blood sugar, such as the involvement of insulin, the glycemic index, and other factors.

3. The Impacts of Blood Sugar on Health: This section investigates the short- and long-term impacts of blood sugar imbalances on a variety of health factors, including energy levels, mood, and chronic diseases.

4. Identifying Blood Sugar Imbalances: Discover the symptoms of high and low blood sugar, diagnostic tests, and how to successfully monitor your blood sugar levels.

5. Nutrition for Blood Sugar Balance: Learn about the benefits of eating a well-balanced diet, how different macronutrients affect blood sugar, and how to plan meals and prepare foods.

6. Lifestyle Changes for Blood Sugar Control: Investigate the impact of exercise, stress management, sleep, and other lifestyle factors on maintaining stable blood sugar levels.

7. Supplements and Natural Remedies: This section discusses critical vitamins, minerals, and herbal supplements that can help manage blood sugar.

8. Special Considerations: Learn how to manage blood sugar for special illnesses like diabetes, hormonal health, and various age groups.

9. Creating Your Personalized Blood Sugar Plan: Create a customized plan to achieve and maintain balanced blood sugar, including setting goals, tracking progress, and establishing a support system.

10. Success Stories and Testimonials: Read about real-life examples of people who have successfully managed their blood sugar and improved their health.

11. The Future of Blood Sugar Management: Discover the most recent advances, technologies, and research in blood sugar monitoring and therapy.

How do I read this book?

You can read this book from cover to cover or go right to the portions that interest you the most. Each chapter is self-contained, providing useful information and practical recommendations that you can use right now.

For Beginners: If you are new to the notion of blood sugar regulation, begin with the fundamental chapters to gain an understanding before progressing to more complex topics.

For experienced readers: If you have a prior understanding of blood sugar management, feel free to jump ahead to the sections that address your special interests or concerns.

Practical tips and action steps

Throughout the book, you will find useful ideas and actionable steps to help you use the information in your daily life. These actionable insights are intended to be straightforward and attainable, making it easier for you to make positive changes and experience results.

Brief ideas: Each chapter contains brief ideas and suggestions for simple blood sugar management measures.

Case Studies: Real-life case studies and success stories are used to demonstrate the effectiveness of the tactics described, as well as to inspire and motivate readers.

Checklists and Worksheets: Use the checklists and worksheets provided to keep track of your progress, set goals, and develop custom plans.

Additional resources

The appendices include a dictionary of words, a list of resources for further study, a recipe index, and an author's comment. These supplementary resources are intended to support your journey and give you the tools and information you require to succeed.

Glossary of Terms: The glossary provides definitions for essential terms and concepts relevant to blood sugar management.

Resources and Further Reading: Learn more about blood sugar and health by reading recommended books, articles, and websites.

Recipe Index: Find a variety of blood sugar-friendly recipes to help you plan healthy and delicious meals.

Author's Note: Discover the author's personal insights and experiences with blood sugar management and health.

Staying motivated and committed

Achieving and maintaining balanced blood sugar levels requires a long-term commitment, and keeping motivated might be difficult at times. Throughout the book, you'll receive motivation and practical tips to keep you on track and conquer challenges.

Setting Realistic Goals: Discover how to set attainable goals and celebrate your accomplishments along the way.

Creating a Support System: Recognize the value of having a support system, whether it is family, friends, or a healthcare professional, to keep you motivated and accountable.

Overcoming hurdles: recognize typical issues

and hurdles to blood sugar management and develop solutions to overcome them.

Using this book as a guide will provide you with the knowledge, tools, and drive you need to regulate your blood sugar and reclaim your health. The "Glucose Revolution" is about more than just controlling blood sugar levels; it is about changing your life and achieving peak health and well-being.

As you embark on this path, remember that little, persistent changes can result in major health improvements. Stay devoted, be patient with yourself, and enjoy every step forward. Welcome to the "Glucose Revolution"; your journey to a better, more vibrant life begins here.

Chapter 1

Understanding Glucose and Blood Sugar

What is glucose?

Glucose is a simple sugar, or monosaccharide, that is used as a fundamental building block of carbohydrates. It is an essential energy source for all living things, including humans. Chemically, glucose is made up of six carbon atoms, twelve hydrogen atoms, and six oxygen atoms, giving it the formula $C_6H_{12}O_6$. This structure makes glucose extremely soluble in water, making it easily transported via the bloodstream.

Glucose can appear in a variety of ways in human diets. It can be found in carbohydrate-rich meals such as fruits, vegetables, cereals, and milk. Once ingested, enzymes in the digestive tract convert these carbs into glucose and other simple sugars. Glucose is then taken into the bloodstream and made accessible for use by the body's cells.

The basic function of glucose is to give energy. Cellular respiration is the mechanism by which cells turn glucose into adenosine triphosphate (ATP). ATP is commonly known as the cell's "energy currency" since it powers a variety of cellular operations such as muscular contraction, nerve impulse transmission, and chemical synthesis. Without a consistent supply of glucose, these important activities would stop, resulting in serious health repercussions.

The role of blood sugar in the body

Blood sugar, often known as blood glucose, is the concentration of glucose in the blood. The body tightly regulates this quantity of glucose to ensure that cells have a continual supply of energy. Maintaining blood sugar levels within a limited range is critical for overall health since both extreme high and low levels can cause serious complications.

The basic function of blood sugar is to provide energy to the cells. After eating, glucose levels in the blood rise as the digested food is absorbed. This causes the pancreas to release insulin, a hormone that aids in the uptake of glucose by cells, especially muscle and liver cells. When glucose enters the cells, it is either used immediately for energy or stored for later use.

Muscle cells store glucose in the form of glycogen, which can be rapidly mobilized during severe physical exercise. Similarly, the liver stores glycogen and serves as a glucose reservoir, releasing glucose into the bloodstream during fasting or in between meals to maintain blood sugar levels. This process ensures that the brain, which relies heavily on glucose for energy, has a steady supply.

Aside from producing energy, glucose participates in a variety of other physiological functions. It is a precursor to the synthesis of essential biomolecules such as nucleotides (the building blocks of DNA and RNA) and lipids. Furthermore, glucose plays a role in the formation of reducing equivalents such as NADPH, which are required for a variety of biosynthetic activities as well as the antioxidant state of cells.

How blood sugar levels are regulated

Blood sugar management is a complex process that involves numerous hormones and organs, most notably the pancreas, liver, and skeletal muscles. This regulation system is intended to keep blood glucose levels within a limited range despite variations in dietary intake and energy expenditure. The pancreas produces the primary hormones involved in blood sugar regulation: insulin and glucagon.

1. Insulin: The Key Regulator.

Insulin is a peptide hormone produced by beta cells in the pancreatic islets. It helps to reduce blood glucose levels by facilitating glucose uptake into cells. When blood glucose levels increase after a meal, insulin is released into the bloodstream. Insulin attaches to receptors on cell surfaces, activating a series of signaling pathways that lead to the insertion of glucose transporters (such as GLUT4) into the cell membrane. These transporters allow glucose to enter the cell, where it can be converted into energy or stored as glycogen.

Insulin promotes glucose uptake while also inhibiting glycogen breakdown (glycogenolysis) and glucose manufacture (gluconeogenesis) in the liver. This dual action ensures that glucose is eliminated from the bloodstream and properly stored, preventing hyperglycemia (excess blood sugar).

2. Glucagon: The Counter-Regulator.

The pancreatic islets' alpha cells also create glucagon, a peptide hormone. Its principal function is to raise blood glucose levels by stimulating the release of glucose from body storage sites. When blood glucose levels fall, such as during a fast or between meals, glucagon is released into the bloodstream. Glucagon increases glycogenolysis in the liver, which converts glycogen into glucose and releases it into the bloodstream.

Furthermore, glucagon promotes gluconeogenesis, which is the creation of glucose from non-carbohydrate sources such as amino acids and glycerol. This process is especially crucial during lengthy periods of fasting or strenuous physical activity, when glycogen levels are low. Glucagon increases the availability of glucose, ensuring that essential organs, particularly the brain, receive an appropriate energy supply.

3. Other Hormones and Factors

While insulin and glucagon are the principal regulators of blood sugar, other hormones and variables play important roles. This includes:

adrenaline (adrenaline): The adrenal glands produce adrenaline in reaction to stress or low blood sugar, which increases glycogenolysis and gluconeogenesis, hence boosting blood glucose levels.

Cortisol, another hormone generated by the adrenal glands, is released during stress and increases gluconeogenesis. It also decreases glucose uptake by specific tissues, ensuring that more glucose is available in the bloodstream.

Growth Hormone: The pituitary gland produces growth hormone, which raises blood glucose levels by stimulating gluconeogenesis and decreasing cell sensitivity to insulin.

Incretins: These are hormones produced by the gut in response to dietary consumption. They increase insulin secretion while inhibiting glucagon release, which helps to manage blood sugar levels after meals.

4. Feedback Mechanisms

Blood sugar levels are regulated through complicated feedback mechanisms that require regular monitoring and correction. These systems keep blood glucose levels within a healthy range.

Negative Feedback Loop: When blood glucose levels rise, the pancreas releases insulin, which reduces blood sugar by promoting glucose uptake and storage. As blood glucose levels drop, insulin output reduces, preventing hypoglycemia. When blood glucose levels fall, the pancreas secretes glucagon, which elevates blood sugar by stimulating glucose release from the liver. This negative feedback loop regulates blood sugar levels.

Glucose Sensing by the Pancreas: The pancreas' beta cells are equipped with glucose sensors that detect changes in blood glucose levels. When glucose levels rise, these sensors stimulate insulin release. When glucose levels fall, insulin secretion is reduced and glucagon release is enhanced. This precise sensing mechanism enables quick and appropriate reactions to changes in blood sugar.

Understanding glucose and blood sugar is essential for comprehending how the body regulates energy and maintains general health. Glucose is an important energy source, and its control is critical for appropriate physiological function. The body painstakingly maintains blood sugar levels using hormones like insulin and glucagon, ensuring that cells receive a consistent supply of energy while minimizing the damaging effects of excessively high or low blood glucose.

Chapter 2

The Science of Blood Sugar.

Balanced blood sugar is essential for general health, influencing energy levels, mood, and long-term well-being. Understanding the science of blood sugar entails digging into the complexities of insulin, the glycemic index, and the different factors that affect blood sugar levels. This chapter will go over these subjects in depth, providing a thorough explanation of how blood sugar works and how to properly manage it.

Insulin and Its Function

Insulin is a hormone made by the pancreas, primarily beta cells in the islets of Langerhans. It helps regulate blood sugar levels by facilitating glucose uptake into the body's cells. When we consume carbs, they are converted into glucose, which enters our bloodstream. An increase in blood glucose levels causes the pancreas to release insulin.

The Role of Insulin:

1. Glucose Uptake: Insulin binds to insulin receptors on cell surfaces, notably muscle and fat cells, prompting them to absorb glucose from the blood. This mechanism reduces blood glucose levels and gives cells the energy they require to function.

2. Storage of Glucose: In addition to aiding glucose uptake, insulin stimulates the storage of excess glucose in the liver and muscles as glycogen. This glycogen can be turned back into glucose when the body needs energy between meals or during physical exertion.

3. Insulin regulates fat metabolism. It slows fat breakdown while promoting fat accumulation in adipose tissue. When insulin levels rise, the body stores more fat, which can lead to weight gain if not balanced with physical exercise.

4. Insulin enhances protein synthesis by increasing the absorption of amino acids into cells. This is critical for muscle growth and repair, making insulin a necessary hormone for total tissue growth and maintenance.

Insulin Resistance and its Implications:

Insulin resistance occurs when cells lose responsiveness to insulin, forcing the pancreas to produce more insulin to accomplish the same impact. This can eventually progress to type 2 diabetes if the pancreas is unable to meet the increasing demand for insulin.

Factors that contribute to insulin resistance include:

Obesity: Excess fat, particularly visceral fat around the abdomen, is strongly associated with insulin resistance.

Physical Inactivity: A lack of regular exercise can diminish insulin's efficiency in stimulating glucose uptake by muscle cells.

Poor Diet: A diet high in processed sugars and unhealthy fats might lead to insulin resistance.

Genetics: Family history and genetic

susceptibility can potentially contribute to the development of insulin resistance.

Managing insulin levels through diet, exercise, and lifestyle modifications is critical for maintaining blood sugar balance and avoiding the development of insulin resistance and type 2 diabetes.

The Glycemic Index Explained

The glycemic index (GI) is a numerical scale that indicates how rapidly and significantly a carbohydrate-containing diet elevates blood glucose levels when compared to a reference food, which is commonly glucose or white bread. Foods are rated on a scale of 0 to 100, with higher scores suggesting a faster and more significant increase in blood glucose levels.

Understanding the glycemic index:
1. High-GI foods: foods with a GI of 70 or above produce a quick increase in blood glucose levels. Examples include white bread, rice, and sweet

snacks. These foods are frequently refined and processed, missing fiber, which delays glucose absorption.

2. Medium-GI Foods: Foods with a GI of 56–69 have a moderate effect on blood glucose levels. Whole wheat bread, sweet potatoes, and some fruits, such as bananas, are other examples.

3. Low-GI Foods: Foods with a GI of 55 or lower encourage blood glucose levels to rise slowly and gradually. The majority of vegetables, legumes, and whole grains, such as barley and quinoa, are good examples. These meals are often high in fiber, which aids in glucose absorption.

Benefits of Low-GI Foods:

Constant Blood Sugar Levels: Eating low-GI foods helps to keep blood sugar levels constant, avoiding the dramatic spikes and decreases associated with high-GI foods. This stability is especially advantageous to people with diabetes or insulin resistance.

Longer Satiety: Low-GI foods keep you feeling fuller for longer, lowering your chances of overeating and aiding in weight management.

Lower Risk of Chronic Diseases: Diets high in low-GI foods are linked to a lower risk of acquiring chronic diseases such as type 2 diabetes, cardiovascular disease, and cancer.

Factors influencing the glycemic index:

A variety of factors can influence a food's glycemic index, including:

Processing: A food's GI tends to increase when it is processed. Whole-grain bread has a lower GI than white bread.

Ripeness: Ripe fruits have a higher GI than unripe fruits because the sugar content rises as the fruit ripens.

Cooking Method: Different cooking procedures might vary a food's GI. For example, pasta cooked al dente has a lower GI than pasta cooked until it is extremely mushy.

Food Combination: The GI of a meal can be modified by the meals eaten together. Adding protein, fat, or fiber to a high-GI diet can reduce the overall GI of the meal.

Factors influencing blood sugar levels:

A variety of factors influence blood sugar levels, including diet, physical activity, hormones, and individual health issues. Understanding these characteristics is vital for optimal blood sugar management.

Dietary factors:
1. Carbohydrate kind and amount: The kind and amount of carbs taken directly affect blood sugar levels. Simple carbs, such as those found in sugary drinks and sweets, are easily digested and absorbed, resulting in rapid blood sugar fluctuations. Complex carbs, including those found in whole grains and vegetables, breakdown more slowly, causing blood sugar levels to gradually rise.

2. Meal Timing and Frequency: Eating regular meals and snacks can help keep blood sugar levels constant. Skipping meals or leaving large gaps between meals can cause blood sugar to plummet, resulting in cravings and overeating later.

3. Fiber Content: Fiber-rich foods decrease

digestion and glucose absorption, resulting in more stable blood sugar levels. Fiber-rich meals such as vegetables, fruits, legumes, and whole grains can help manage your blood sugar levels.

4. Protein and Fat: Including protein and healthy fats in your meals will help decrease glucose absorption and minimize blood sugar increases. Protein and fat help promote a sense of fullness, which reduces the chance of overeating.

Physical Activity:

Regular physical activity helps to control blood sugar levels by raising insulin sensitivity and stimulating glucose absorption by muscle cells. Different types of exercise, such as aerobic exercise (walking, jogging, and cycling) and resistance training (weightlifting), can help with blood sugar management. Consistency is essential; even moderate movement on a daily basis can improve blood sugar management significantly.

Hormonal Factors:

Several hormones, in addition to insulin, affect blood sugar levels:

Glucagon: The pancreas produces glucagon, which elevates blood sugar levels by prompting the liver to convert stored glycogen to glucose and release it into the bloodstream.

Cortisol, often known as the stress hormone, can raise blood sugar levels by boosting gluconeogenesis, which is the liver's creation of glucose from non-carbohydrate sources. Chronic stress and raised cortisol levels can lead to excessive blood sugar and insulin resistance.

Epinephrine (adrenaline): Released during stress or activity, epinephrine raises blood sugar levels by activating the liver to produce glucose and decreasing insulin's efficacy.

Individual Health Conditions:

1. Diabetes: Types 1 and 2 have a direct impact on blood sugar management. In type 1 diabetes, the immune system assaults and destroys insulin-producing beta cells in the pancreas, resulting in an absolute insulin shortage. Type 2 diabetes occurs when the body becomes insulin resistant and the pancreas is unable to produce enough insulin to overcome this resistance.

2. Metabolic syndrome is a group of diseases that include high blood pressure, high blood sugar, extra abdominal fat, and abnormal cholesterol levels, all of which raise the risk of heart disease, stroke, and type 2 diabetes. Managing metabolic syndrome entails treating each of these disorders with lifestyle changes and, if necessary, medicines.

3. Polycystic Ovary Syndrome (PCOS) is a hormonal condition that affects many women of reproductive age. It is linked to insulin resistance, which can cause elevated blood sugar levels and an increased risk of developing type 2 diabetes.

Other factors:

1. Sleep: Poor sleep quality and insufficient sleep might have a negative impact on blood sugar levels and insulin sensitivity. Establishing a consistent sleep schedule and getting enough sleep are critical for maintaining healthy blood sugar levels.

2. Certain drugs have been shown to have an effect on blood sugar levels. Corticosteroids, for

example, can cause blood sugar levels to rise. It is critical to address any potential side effects with your healthcare professional.

3. Hydration: Staying hydrated promotes healthy blood sugar levels. Dehydration can raise blood sugar levels by decreasing blood volume and raising the quantity of glucose in the bloodstream.

Monitor and manage blood sugar levels:

Blood sugar management requires regular monitoring and intelligent lifestyle decisions. Here are a few strategies:

Regular Monitoring: Using a blood glucose meter, check your blood sugar levels on a regular basis. This explains how various foods, activities, and stressors affect your blood sugar.

Healthy Eating: Maintain a well-balanced diet rich in nutrient-dense foods. Choose low-GI foods, add fiber and protein,

Consume healthy fats and avoid sugary and highly processed foods.

Physical Activity: Aim for at least 150 minutes of moderate aerobic activity or 75 minutes of strenuous activity per week, with muscle-strengthening activities on two or more days per week.

Stress Management: Use stress-reduction practices like mindfulness, meditation, yoga, or deep breathing exercises to help control cortisol levels and keep blood sugar constant.

Adequate Sleep: Prioritize sleep by sticking to a regular sleep schedule, providing a relaxing sleep environment, and aiming for 7-9 hours of quality sleep per night.

Understanding the science of blood sugar is critical for anyone hoping to recover their health through controlled blood sugar levels. Understanding the responsibilities of insulin, the glycemic index, and the numerous factors that influence blood sugar can allow you to make informed decisions and adopt effective strategies for maintaining optimal health.

Chapter 3

The Effect of Blood Sugar on Health.

The short-term effects of blood sugar spikes

Blood sugar, or glucose, is an essential source of energy for the body's cells. However, abrupt spikes in blood sugar levels can cause a range of short-term physiological repercussions. These spikes, which are frequently triggered by the consumption of high-glycemic foods, stress, or other circumstances, can upset the body's balance and elicit instant reactions.

1. Energy CrashesOne of the most obvious short-term consequences of blood sugar rises is an energy collapse. When you eat meals heavy in refined sugars or simple carbohydrates, like candy, soda, or white bread, your blood sugar

levels can skyrocket. In reaction, the pancreas secretes a considerable amount of insulin to aid in glucose uptake into cells. This rapid insulin response can cause blood sugar levels to drop dramatically, resulting in weariness, irritation, and problems concentrating. These energy collapses can set off a vicious cycle in which people consume more sugary meals to battle low energy, prolonging the pattern of spikes and crashes.

2. Increased hungerBlood sugar increases can also affect appetite and hunger levels. High insulin levels, caused by a blood sugar surge, can lead to increased appetite and cravings for sugary or carbohydrate-rich foods. This occurrence, known as "reactive hypoglycemia," occurs when the body overcompensates for the initial rise, resulting in low blood sugar levels that cause the brain to crave more food. As a result, individuals may develop a pattern of overeating and weight gain, complicating blood sugar regulation.

3. Mood swings and cognitive impairmentsA continuous supply of glucose is critical for the brain's optimal function. Blood sugar increases, followed by fast reductions, can impair cognitive function and mood regulation. Symptoms could include mood changes, anxiety, and difficulties concentrating. For example, after eating a high-sugar meal, one may experience a surge of energy and exhilaration, followed by a period of lethargy and irritation as blood sugar levels drop. This variability has a negative influence on productivity, emotional well-being, and overall mental health.

4. Temporary Insulin ResistanceFrequent blood sugar rises can cause transient insulin resistance, in which the body's cells become less sensitive to insulin. As the body struggles to maintain normal blood sugar levels, this condition can cause increased levels of glucose and insulin to circulate in the bloodstream. While transitory insulin resistance is a natural physiological reaction, repeated occurrences raise the chance of developing more permanent insulin

resistance, which is a major factor in the development of type 2 diabetes.

Long-term health consequences.

Chronic blood sugar abnormalities have serious long-term health implications. Consistently high blood sugar levels, which are commonly caused by poor food choices, sedentary lifestyles, and other factors, can lead to a variety of major health problems.

1. Type 2 diabetes.One of the most well-known long-term implications of frequent blood sugar increases is the development of type 2 diabetes. This syndrome develops when the body grows resistant to insulin, resulting in high blood sugar levels over time. Prolonged insulin resistance can fatigue the pancreas, reducing its ability to produce enough insulin. As a result, people with type 2 diabetes must control their blood sugar levels with medicine, food, and lifestyle changes to avoid future complications.

2. Cardiovascular diseaseChronically high blood sugar levels can harm blood vessels and raise the risk of cardiovascular disease. Elevated glucose levels can promote inflammation and contribute to the formation of plaque in the arteries, resulting in atherosclerosis. This disorder narrows and hardens the arteries, increasing the likelihood of a heart attack, stroke, or other cardiovascular event. Furthermore, excessive blood sugar levels can raise blood pressure and cholesterol, increasing the risk of heart disease.

3. NeuropathyLong-term blood sugar abnormalities can damage the nerve system, causing neuropathy. Diabetic neuropathy, in particular, is a typical side effect of chronic high blood sugar levels. It can cause symptoms including numbness, tingling, and pain, which commonly begin in the hands and feet. In severe situations, neuropathy can impair the digestive system, heart, and other organs, resulting in considerable disability and a lower quality of life.

4. Kidney damageThe kidneys perform a critical role in removing waste from the circulation. Chronic high blood sugar levels can harm the kidneys' tiny blood capillaries, reducing their ability to operate correctly. This illness, known as diabetic nephropathy, can lead to kidney failure if not properly controlled. People with renal impairment may need dialysis or a kidney transplant to survive.

5. Vision ProblemsHigh blood sugar levels can also damage the blood vessels in the eyes, causing diabetic retinopathy. If not addressed, this illness can cause blurred vision, floaters, and possibly blindness. Regular eye exams and blood sugar management are critical for avoiding and treating diabetic retinopathy.

The Relationship Between Blood Sugar and Chronic Disease

The link between blood sugar and chronic diseases goes beyond diabetes. Elevated blood sugar levels and insulin resistance are linked to a variety of other chronic health issues, emphasizing the necessity of maintaining stable blood sugar levels for overall health.

1. ObesityObesity is closely associated with insulin resistance and elevated blood sugar levels. Excess body fat, especially around the abdomen, might increase insulin resistance, making it more difficult for the body to control blood sugar levels. Furthermore, elevated blood sugar and insulin levels can encourage fat storage, triggering a feedback loop that exacerbates weight gain and obesity. Obesity is a risk factor for a variety of chronic conditions, including heart disease, stroke, and several malignancies.

2. Metabolic SyndromeMetabolic syndrome is a collection of disorders that occur together and raise the risk of heart disease, stroke, and type 2 diabetes. These disorders include excessive blood pressure, high blood sugar, extra abdominal fat, and abnormal cholesterol or triglyceride levels. Insulin resistance and chronic

high blood sugar levels are crucial to the development of metabolic syndrome; hence, blood sugar management is critical for avoiding and treating the condition.

3. Inflammatory conditions.Chronic high blood sugar levels can lead to systemic inflammation, which is a common underlying cause of many chronic diseases. Inflammation can harm tissues and organs, resulting in arthritis, cardiovascular disease, and some types of cancer. Individuals who maintain regulated blood sugar levels can help minimize inflammation and lower their chance of acquiring certain inflammatory disorders.

4. Cognitive decline with Alzheimer's diseaseRecent research indicates a clear link between blood sugar levels and cognitive impairment. High blood sugar and insulin resistance have been linked to an increased risk of Alzheimer's disease and other types of dementia. Alzheimer's disease has even been dubbed "type 3 diabetes" by some experts due to the function of insulin resistance in the brain.

Managing blood sugar levels may therefore be a key technique for maintaining cognitive function and preventing neurodegenerative disorders.

5. Polycystic Ovarian Syndrome (PCOS)PCOS is a hormonal illness that affects women of reproductive age. It is characterized by irregular menstrual periods, elevated androgen levels, and polycystic ovaries. Insulin resistance is a major contributor to PCOS, as high insulin levels can exacerbate hormonal imbalances and increase the likelihood of developing the illness. Women with PCOS must manage their blood sugar levels in order to regulate their menstrual cycles, minimize symptoms, and increase fertility.

Chapter 4

Determining Blood Sugar Imbalances

Identifying and understanding blood sugar abnormalities is critical for sustaining good health. Blood sugar, or glucose levels, have a profound impact on how our bodies function, affecting everything from energy levels to cognitive function and overall well-being. This chapter will look at the symptoms of high and low blood sugar, the diagnostic tests and monitoring tools available, and how to interpret blood sugar readings.

Symptoms of High or Low Blood Sugar

High blood sugar (hyperglycemia).

Hyperglycemia occurs when there is an excess of glucose in the bloodstream. This can be attributed to a variety of circumstances, including insufficient insulin synthesis, insulin resistance, or an excessive carbohydrate intake. Recognizing the signs of high blood sugar is critical for early intervention and control.

1. Increased Urination (Polyuria): One of the first indications of hyperglycemia is excessive urination. The kidneys remove excess glucose from the bloodstream by filtering it through urine.

2. Increased thirst (Polydipsia): Frequent urine causes the body to lose a substantial amount of water, resulting in dehydration. This causes acute thirst as the body tries to restore lost fluids.

3. exhaustion: High blood sugar levels can impair the body's ability to use glucose for

energy, resulting in persistent exhaustion and weakness.

4. Blurred Vision: High glucose levels can cause the lenses of the eyes to expand, resulting in blurred vision. This symptom usually goes away after blood sugar levels return to normal.

5. Headaches: Fluctuations in blood sugar levels can cause headaches, which may range from mild to severe.

6. Unintended Weight Loss: Even if they eat normally or more, people with high blood sugar may lose weight for no apparent reason. This happens when the body is unable to correctly use glucose and starts breaking down muscle and fat for energy.

7. Slow Healing of Cuts and Wounds: High glucose levels can hinder the body's natural healing processes, resulting in longer recovery periods for cuts, bruises, and infections.

8. Recurrent Infections: High blood sugar levels can impair the immune system, leaving the body

more vulnerable to infections, especially urinary tract infections and skin infections.

9. Numbness or Tingling in Hands and Feet: Chronic high blood sugar levels can damage nerves, resulting in diabetic neuropathy, which causes numbness, tingling, and discomfort in the extremities.

Low blood sugar (hypoglycemia).

Hypoglycemia occurs when blood sugar levels fall below 70 mg/dL. This illness can be very deadly if not treated rapidly, as glucose is the brain's principal energy supply. Recognizing the signs of low blood sugar is crucial for taking appropriate action.

1. Shakiness: One of the most prevalent symptoms of hypoglycemia is a sensation of shakiness or tremors, particularly in the hands.

2. Perspiration: Excessive perspiration, especially when not coupled with physical activity or high temperatures, might be an indication of low blood sugar.

3. Hunger: Severe hunger, particularly a desire for sweet meals, may indicate that blood sugar levels are declining.

4. Irritability: Hypoglycemia can influence mood, resulting in feelings of irritability, anxiety, or agitation.

5. exhaustion: Similar to hyperglycemia, low blood sugar can also create sensations of exhaustion and weakness due to the body's inability to obtain sufficient energy.

6. Confusion: As glucose levels drop, cognitive function might become affected, leading to confusion, trouble concentrating, and memory difficulties.

7. Dizziness or Lightheadedness: Low blood sugar can produce dizziness or lightheadedness, which can be especially dangerous if it results in falls or accidents.

8. Palpitations are rapid or irregular heartbeats that occur when blood sugar levels are low.

9. Blurred vision: Like hyperglycemia, hypoglycemia can cause visual problems, including blurred vision.

10. Hypoglycemia can cause seizures, loss of consciousness, and even coma if not treated swiftly.

Diagnostic tests and monitoring tools

Accurate diagnosis and monitoring of blood sugar levels are critical for controlling blood sugar abnormalities. Individuals and healthcare providers can use a variety of tests and tools to monitor glucose levels and make informed decisions regarding treatment and lifestyle changes.

Blood glucose tests

1. The Fasting Blood Glucose Test checks blood sugar levels after an individual has fasted for at least 8 hours. It is usually conducted in the morning, before breakfast. Normal fasting blood

glucose levels range between 70 and 99 mg/dL. Values between 100 and 125 mg/dL indicate prediabetes, whereas values above 126 mg/dL indicate diabetes.

2. The Oral Glucose Tolerance Test (OGTT) assesses how efficiently the body handles glucose. After fasting, an individual takes a glucose-rich beverage, and blood sugar levels are tested at regular intervals over the next two hours. Normal readings are less than 140 mg/dL; prediabetes is defined as levels between 140 and 199 mg/dL; and diabetes is defined as values of 200 mg/dL or more.

3. The hemoglobin A1c (HbA1c) test calculates an average of blood sugar levels over the previous two to three months by detecting the proportion of glucose linked to hemoglobin in the blood. Normal HbA1c values are less than 5.7%; prediabetes is defined as levels between 5.7% and 6.4%; and diabetes is defined as levels of 6.5% or higher.

4. Random Blood Glucose Test: This test measures blood sugar levels throughout the day, regardless of when the individual last ate. A result of 200 mg/dL or greater indicates diabetes, especially if accompanied by hyperglycemic symptoms.

Continuous glucose monitoring (CGM).

Continuous glucose monitoring (CGM) systems track blood sugar levels in real time, all day and night. A tiny sensor is implanted under the skin, usually on the belly or upper arm, to test glucose levels in the interstitial fluid. The sensor delivers data to a monitor or smartphone app, allowing users to see trends and patterns in their blood glucose levels. CGM devices are especially beneficial for diabetics who need to closely monitor their glucose levels and make changes to their diet, activity, or medications.

Self-monitoring of blood glucose (SMBG)

Self-monitoring of blood glucose (SMBG) is using a blood glucose meter to assess blood sugar levels at particular times of day. Individuals pierce their finger to collect a little blood sample, which is then placed on a test strip and inserted into the meter for a reading. SMBG enables people to monitor their blood sugar levels, make smart food and activity choices, and change their medication as appropriate. It is an effective strategy for treating hyperglycemia and hypoglycemia.

Understand your blood sugar numbers.

Interpreting blood sugar data is critical for efficiently managing blood sugar levels and making informed food, exercise, and medication choices. Understanding what varied blood sugar readings signify can help people take the necessary steps to preserve good health.

Normal blood sugar levels.

Fasting blood glucose: 70 to 99 mg/dLPostprandial blood glucose (1-2 hours after eating): <140 mg/dLHbA1c is less than 5.7%.

Prediabetes

Prediabetes is a condition in which blood sugar levels exceed normal but are not high enough to be classified as diabetes. It indicates that an individual is at a higher risk of developing type 2 diabetes and other health issues.

Fasting blood glucose: 100 to 125 mg/dLPostprandial blood glucose: 140–199 mg/dLHbA1c: 5.7–6.4%

Diabetes

Diabetes is diagnosed when blood sugar levels are consistently high and the body fails to control glucose adequately. There are two forms of diabetes: type 1 and type 2.

Fasting blood glucose is 126 mg/dL or above.Postprandial blood glucose: 200 mg/dL or more.HbA1c of 6.5% or above.

Target blood sugar levels for people with diabetes

Maintaining target blood sugar levels is critical for diabetics to avoid complications and preserve good overall health. These goal ranges may vary depending on individual health problems and healthcare practitioners' recommendations.

Fasting blood glucose: 80 to 130 mg/dLPostprandial blood glucose is less than 180 mg/dL.HbA1c: less than 7% (individual objectives may differ).

Factors affecting blood sugar levels

Blood sugar levels can be influenced by a variety of circumstances; therefore, it is critical to keep this in mind when interpreting results and making lifestyle changes.

1. Diet: The types and quantities of foods eaten have a major impact on blood sugar levels. Carbohydrates, for example, convert quickly to glucose, causing blood sugar to rise.

2. Exercise reduces blood sugar levels by increasing insulin sensitivity and enhancing glucose absorption by muscles.

3. Medication: Blood sugar levels are managed using drugs such as insulin and oral hypoglycemic agents. It is critical to adhere to prescribed dosages and timetables.

4. Stress: Physical and emotional stress can raise blood sugar levels by causing the production of stress hormones.

5. Ill

Acute or chronic illnesses might have an impact on blood sugar regulation, necessitating dietary or pharmacological changes.

6. Sleep: Poor sleep quality or insufficient sleep might impair blood sugar management and insulin sensitivity.

Tips to Manage Blood Sugar Levels

Effective blood sugar management requires a combination of monitoring, lifestyle adjustments, and, in some situations, medication. Here are some methods to help keep blood sugar balanced:

1. Monitor regularly: Use SMBG or CGM to measure blood sugar levels and spot patterns or trends.

2. Eat Balanced Meals: Focus on a diet rich in whole grains, lean proteins, healthy fats, and plenty of fruits and vegetables. Avoid consuming too much sugar or processed meals.

3. Stay Active: Build physical activity into your daily routine, aiming for at least 150 minutes of moderate exercise per week.

4. Manage stress: Try stress-reduction practices like mindfulness, meditation, yoga, or deep breathing exercises.

5. Get Adequate Sleep: Aim for 7-9 hours of quality sleep per night to promote general health and blood sugar management.

6. Follow Medication Guidelines: Take drugs as prescribed by your healthcare professional and report any adverse effects or concerns.

7. Stay Hydrated: Drink plenty of water throughout the day to improve overall health and help keep blood sugar constant.

8. Plan Ahead: Keep snacks on hand, remain hydrated, and be aware of any triggers that may alter your blood sugar levels.

Individuals can manage their blood sugar levels more successfully by knowing the signs of blood sugar imbalances, using diagnostic tests and monitoring tools, and interpreting blood sugar data. This understanding is critical for avoiding issues, enhancing general health, and regaining control of one's well-being.

Chapter 5

Nutrition and Blood Sugar Balance

The importance of a balanced diet.

A balanced diet is essential for maintaining good health and well-being. It is even more important when maintaining blood sugar levels, which are necessary for avoiding and controlling illnesses such as diabetes, metabolic syndrome, and other health difficulties. A balanced diet not only helps you maintain a healthy weight, but it also ensures that your body gets the nutrients it needs to function properly.

When it comes to blood sugar balance, a balanced diet entails eating a range of foods in the appropriate quantities to maintain a stable blood glucose level. This entails providing the right balance of carbs, proteins, and fats, as well as the necessary vitamins, minerals, and fiber. Each of these nutrients has a distinct role in the way your body metabolizes glucose and regulates energy levels.

Macronutrients and Blood Sugar

Macronutrients—carbohydrates, proteins, and fats—make up the majority of our diet and have a direct impact on blood sugar levels.

1. Carbs.

Carbohydrates are the body's primary source of energy, but they have the greatest impact on blood glucose levels. When you ingest carbs, your body converts them into glucose, which circulates in your bloodstream. The glycemic index (GI) is a method for determining how rapidly a carbohydrate-rich food elevates blood glucose levels. Foods with a high GI induce sudden blood sugar increases, whereas foods with a foods with a low GI generate a slower, more steady increase.

Types of Carbohydrates:

Simple carbohydrates are sugars present in fruits, milk, and sweetened foods. They are easily absorbed and can produce high blood sugar levels.

Complex Carbohydrates: Found in whole grains, legumes, and vegetables, these are absorbed more slowly, causing a gradual rise in blood sugar levels.

2. Proteins.

Proteins are necessary for tissue growth and repair, as well as muscle and organ function. They have little immediate effect on blood sugar levels, but they can alter them indirectly. Including enough protein in your diet slows the absorption of carbohydrates, lowering blood sugar after meals. Furthermore, protein increases satiety, which can help reduce overeating and aid with weight management.

3. Fats

Fats provide critical energy and are required for the absorption of fat-soluble vitamins (A, D, E, and K). While lipids do not directly alter blood sugar, they do play an important role in overall metabolic health. Avocados, nuts, seeds, and olive oil include healthy fats, which can help increase insulin sensitivity. However, trans fats and saturated fats should be avoided or limited because they might contribute to insulin resistance and other health complications.

Superfoods to Stabilize Blood Sugar

Because of their nutrient content and health advantages, many foods are especially helpful at regulating blood sugar levels. These superfoods can help you manage your blood sugar:

1. Leafy greens.

Leafy greens such as spinach, kale, and Swiss chard are low in calories and carbs while high in fiber, vitamins, and minerals. They have little effect on blood sugar levels and are high in antioxidants, which can help reduce inflammation and increase insulin sensitivity.

2. Berries

Berries, such as blueberries, strawberries, and raspberries, are rich in fiber and antioxidants. They have a low glycemic index and can boost insulin sensitivity. Berries' antioxidants also help to counteract oxidative stress and inflammation, both of which are associated with insulin resistance.

3. Nuts and seeds.

Almonds, walnuts, chia seeds, and flaxseeds are rich in healthy fats, protein, and fiber. They help decrease glucose absorption, avoiding blood sugar increases. Furthermore, they include critical nutrients such as magnesium, which is required for glucose metabolism.

4. Whole grains

Whole grains, such as quinoa, brown rice, oats, and barley, are high in fiber and have a lower glycemic index than processed grains. The fiber content slows the digestion and absorption of carbohydrates, resulting in more stable blood sugar levels. Whole grains also supply critical vitamins and minerals, such as B vitamins and magnesium.

5. Legumes

Legumes, including beans, lentils, and chickpeas, are abundant in protein, fiber, and complex carbs. They have a low glycemic index and can help control blood sugar levels. Legumes' fiber also enhances intestinal health, which is beneficial to general metabolic health.

6. Cinnamon.

Cinnamon is a spice that has been linked to increased insulin sensitivity and decreased blood sugar levels. Including cinnamon in your diet can improve the flavor of meals while also providing potential blood sugar advantages.

7. Apple cider vinegar.

Apple cider vinegar has been shown to improve insulin sensitivity and reduce blood sugar levels following meals. These advantages can be obtained by including apple cider vinegar in your diet, such as through salad dressings or diluting it with water.

Meal Plans and Recipes

Effective meal planning is essential for maintaining stable blood sugar levels. By organizing your meals and snacks, you can guarantee that you are eating a well-balanced diet rich in macronutrients and superfoods. Here are some meal planning guidelines and dish ideas to help you get started:

Tips for meal planning:

1. Include a Variety of Foods: To ensure balanced nutrition, make sure your meals include a combination of carbohydrates, proteins, and fats.

2. Focus on Fiber: To help regulate blood sugar levels, eat foods high in fiber, such as whole grains, legumes, veggies, and fruits.

3. Keep track of portion sizes to avoid overeating, which can contribute to blood sugar rises.

4. Eat Regularly: To keep your blood sugar constant, eat modest, balanced meals and snacks throughout the day.

5. Stay Hydrated: Drink enough water.

throughout the day to stay hydrated and maintain good health.

Recipe Ideas:

1. Breakfast: Berry Chia Seed Pudding

Ingredients:

2 tablespoons of chia seeds

1 cup unsweetened almond milk

1 teaspoon of vanilla extract

1/2 cup mixed berries

1 tablespoon chopped nuts (optional)

Stevia or honey to taste (optional)

Instructions:

1. In a bowl, mix chia seeds, almond milk, and vanilla extract.

2. Let it sit for at least 30 minutes or overnight in the refrigerator until it thickens.

3. Top with mixed berries and chopped nuts before serving.

4. Sweeten with stevia or honey, if desired.

2. Lunch: Quinoa and Black Bean Salad

Ingredients:

1 cup cooked quinoa

1 can of black beans, rinsed and drained

1 cup cherry tomatoes, halved

1 avocado, diced

1/4 cup red onion, finely chopped

2 tablespoons fresh cilantro, chopped

Juice of 1 lime

2 tablespoons of olive oil

Salt and pepper to taste

Instructions:

1. In a large bowl, combine cooked quinoa, black beans, cherry tomatoes, avocado, red onion, and cilantro.

2. In a small bowl, whisk together lime juice, olive oil, salt, and pepper.

3. Pour the dressing over the quinoa mixture and toss to combine.

4. Serve chilled or at room temperature.

3. Snack: Hummus and Veggie Sticks

Ingredients:

1 can chickpeas, rinsed and drained

1/4 cup tahini

2 tablespoons of olive oil

Juice of 1 lemon

2 cloves of garlic

1/2 teaspoon ground cumin

Salt to taste

Water, as needed

Assorted vegetable sticks (carrots, celery, bell peppers, cucumber)

Instructions:

1. In a food processor, combine chickpeas, tahini, olive oil, lemon juice, garlic, cumin, and salt.

2. Blend until smooth, adding water as needed to reach the desired consistency.

3. Serve with assorted vegetable sticks for dipping.

4. Dinner: Baked Salmon with Roasted Vegetables

Ingredients:

4 salmon fillets

2 tablespoons of olive oil

1 lemon, sliced

2 cloves garlic, minced

1 teaspoon dried dill

Salt and pepper to taste

1 cup of broccoli florets

1 cup of cauliflower florets

1 cup sliced carrots

1 cup Brussels sprouts, halved

Instructions:

1. Preheat the oven to 400°F (200°C).

2. Place salmon fillets on a baking sheet lined with parchment paper.

3. Drizzle with olive oil and top with lemon slices, minced garlic, dried dill, salt, and pepper.

4. Arrange the vegetables around the salmon on the baking sheet.

5. Drizzle the vegetables with olive oil and season with salt and pepper.

6. Bake for 20–25 minutes, or until the salmon is cooked through and the vegetables are tender.

5. Dessert: Greek Yogurt with Nuts and Berries

Ingredients:

1 cup of plain Greek yogurt

1/2 cup mixed berries

2 tablespoons chopped nuts (almonds, walnuts, or pecans)

1 teaspoon honey or stevia (optional)

1/2 teaspoon cinnamon

Instructions:

1. In a bowl, combine Greek yogurt, mixed berries, and chopped nuts.

2. Drizzle with honey or stevia, if desired.

3. Sprinkle with cinnamon before serving.

Chapter 6

Lifestyle Alterations for Blood Sugar Control

Balancing blood sugar is more than just what you eat; it also entails making strategic lifestyle modifications that improve your body's capacity to keep glucose levels stable. This chapter goes into the critical functions of exercise, stress management, sleep, and toxin reduction in blood sugar regulation. By adopting these modifications into your everyday routine, you can dramatically improve your general health and well-being.

The Role of Exercise

Regular physical activity is an essential component of successful blood sugar management. Exercise improves insulin sensitivity, allowing your cells to use available glucose more efficiently. Here's how several types of exercise can improve blood sugar control:

Aerobic exercise.

Aerobic workouts like walking, jogging, swimming, and cycling are extremely beneficial for improving cardiovascular health and increasing insulin sensitivity. Aerobic activity causes your muscles to consume glucose for energy, lowering blood sugar levels. Moderate-intensity aerobic activity, such as brisk walking for at least 30 minutes per day, has been proven in studies to dramatically lower the risk of acquiring type 2 diabetes while also helping to control existing symptoms.

Resistance Training

Resistance training, often known as strength training, is a set of exercises that build muscle strength and mass. This category includes activities such as weightlifting, bodyweight exercises, and resistance band workouts. Building muscle mass raises your resting metabolic rate, which means you burn more calories even when you aren't actively exercising. Furthermore, muscles store glucose as glycogen; therefore, having more muscular mass can help with glucose storage and use, resulting in better blood sugar control.

High-Intensity Interval Training (HIIT)

HIIT consists of short bursts of intensive exercise followed by intervals of rest or low-intensity activity. This kind of training has gained popularity due to its efficiency and effectiveness. HIIT can greatly enhance insulin sensitivity and glucose metabolism, and it often takes less time than standard workout approaches. For example, a typical HIIT workout can consist of 30 seconds of sprinting followed by 1-2 minutes of walking, which is done for 20–30 minutes.

Tips to Incorporate Exercise

1. Set realistic goals: Begin with achievable objectives and progressively raise the intensity and duration of your workouts.
2. Mix It Up: Include a variety of exercises to keep your workout interesting and work different muscle groups.
3. Maintain Consistency: Aim for at least 150 minutes of moderate-intensity aerobic exercise per week, plus two sessions of weight training.
4. Monitor Blood Sugar: If you have diabetes, measure your blood sugar levels before and after exercise to see how different activities influence you.

Stress management techniques

Chronic stress can cause havoc with your blood sugar levels. When you are stressed, your body produces hormones such as cortisol and adrenaline, which can raise blood sugar. Managing stress is thus critical for achieving stable glucose levels. Here are some successful stress management strategies:

Mindfulness and meditation

Mindfulness activities, including meditation, have been demonstrated to reduce stress and improve general health. Focusing on the present moment and noticing your thoughts without judgment might help you relax and lessen the effects of stress on your body. Meditation on a regular basis can help reduce cortisol levels and maintain blood sugar balance.

Deep breathing exercises.

Deep breathing techniques can stimulate the parasympathetic nervous system, promoting relaxation and lowering tension. Simple approaches for stress management include diaphragmatic breathing, which involves inhaling deeply with your nose, holding for a few seconds, and exhaling gently through your mouth.

Physical activity.

Exercise is good for both your physical and mental wellbeing. Endorphins, which are natural mood improvers, are released during physical exertion. Regular exercise can help with anxiety and sadness, both of which can lead to chronic stress.

Yoga and Tai Chi

Yoga and tai chi, which mix physical movement with mindfulness and deep breathing, are great stress-reduction practices. These exercises increase flexibility, strength, and balance while also relaxing the mind and lowering stress hormones.

Time management and organization

Effective time management can help minimize stress by ensuring that you have adequate time for work, rest, and self-care. Key tactics include prioritizing tasks, setting realistic deadlines, and avoiding overcommitment. Planners and digital calendars are useful tools for staying organized and reducing feelings of overwhelm.

The importance of sleep

Sleep is an essential component of good health and has a substantial impact on blood sugar regulation. Poor sleep can cause insulin resistance and elevated blood sugar levels. Here's why healthy sleep is important and how you can enhance your sleep quality:

How Does Sleep Affect Blood Sugar

1. Insulin Sensitivity: Adequate sleep promotes insulin sensitivity. Sleep deprivation, on the other hand, can make your cells more insulin-resistant, resulting in elevated blood sugar levels.

2. Sleep regulates hormones that influence hunger and appetite, such as leptin and ghrelin. Poor sleep might boost appetites for high-sugar

foods, raising blood sugar levels.

3. Stress Reduction: Getting enough sleep lowers cortisol levels, which helps keep blood sugar levels constant.

Tips for improved sleep

1. Establish a Routine: To regulate your body's internal clock, go to bed and get up at the same time every day, even on weekends.

2. Create a Sleep-Friendly Environment: Keep your bedroom dark, quiet, and cool. Invest in a comfy mattress and pillow.

3. Limit Screen Time: Avoid using screens (phones, tablets, and computers) at least an hour before bedtime, as the blue light they emit can disrupt your sleep cycle.

4. Avoid stimulants: Limit your caffeine and nicotine intake, particularly in the hours before bedtime.

5. Relax Before Bed: Create a pre-sleep routine that allows you to unwind, such as reading, having a warm bath, or practicing relaxation techniques.

Reducing toxic exposure

Exposure to environmental pollutants might have an impact on your blood sugar levels and general health. These pollutants can disrupt hormonal balance, promote inflammation, and lead to insulin resistance. Reducing your exposure to toxins is an important step toward maintaining normal blood sugar levels.

Common Toxins: Their Effects

1. Pesticides are found in non-organic fruits and vegetables and can impair endocrine function, contributing to insulin resistance.
2. Heavy metals, such as lead, mercury, and cadmium, can interfere with insulin synthesis and glucose metabolism.
3. Endocrine disruptors: Plastics and personal care items contain chemicals including bisphenol A (BPA) and phthalates, which can mimic hormones and alter metabolic processes.
4. Air Pollution: Polluted air can cause

inflammation and insulin resistance, which can lead to elevated blood sugar levels.

Tips to Reduce Toxin Exposure

1. Eat organic: To decrease your exposure to pesticides, choose organic produce. If organic produce isn't available, carefully wash fruits and vegetables to remove pesticide residue.
2. Filter your water: To eliminate toxins from your drinking water, use a water filter.
3. Avoid Plastic: Limit your usage of plastic containers and wrap, especially when storing food. Choose glass, stainless steel, or BPA-free alternatives.
4. Choose Natural Products: Choose personal care products, cleaning supplies, and household items that do not contain dangerous chemicals.
5. Improve interior air quality: To reduce interior air pollution, use air purifiers, keep indoor plants, and maintain sufficient ventilation.

Integrating Lifestyle Changes for Optimal Blood Sugar Management

Making lifestyle modifications for blood sugar control necessitates a comprehensive strategy. Here's how to successfully merge these changes:

1. Create a complete plan that incorporates regular exercise, stress management techniques, a consistent sleep routine, and toxin-reduction tactics.
2. Set tiny goals: Begin with tiny, doable improvements and progressively increase. For example, start with a 10-minute daily walk and progressively increase the duration and effort.
3. Track Your Progress: Keep a notebook or use an app to record your activities, stress levels, sleep habits, and any changes in blood sugar levels.
4. Stay Motivated: Set realistic goals, celebrate minor accomplishments, and seek help from friends, family, or a support group.
5. Seek Professional Help: Consult a doctor, nutritionist, or personal trainer to personalize

your plan to your specific needs and verify you're on the correct track.

You may control your blood sugar levels and improve your overall health by adopting regular exercise, effective stress management, prioritizing sleep, and limiting your exposure to contaminants. These lifestyle adjustments not only aid with blood sugar management but also lead to a more balanced, healthier, and more satisfying existence.

Chapter 7

Supplements and Natural Remedies.

Dietary and lifestyle modifications are essential in the quest for balanced blood sugar levels, but they can be supplemented with the careful use of vitamins and natural therapies. These can help to alleviate dietary shortages, improve insulin sensitivity, and promote overall metabolic health. This chapter delves into critical vitamins and minerals, herbal supplements for blood sugar regulation, and the significance of probiotics in gut health.

Essential vitamins and minerals

A proper diet is essential for maintaining normal blood sugar levels. Vitamins and minerals have important roles in metabolic processes and insulin regulation. Here are some key foods that can help regulate blood sugar:

Vitamin D

Vitamin D is required for a variety of human activities, including immune system modulation and bone strength. According to research, optimal vitamin D levels are essential for insulin sensitivity and glucose metabolism. Vitamin D deficiency increases the likelihood of insulin resistance and type 2 diabetes.

Sources include sun exposure, fatty fish (such as salmon, mackerel, and sardines), fortified dairy products, and supplements.
Recommended Intake: The recommended daily allowance (RDA) for adults is from 600 to 800 IU; however, greater doses may be required for people with a deficiency, as directed by a doctor.

Magnesium

Magnesium is a mineral that participates in more than 300 biochemical activities, including those related to glucose and insulin metabolism. Adequate magnesium consumption improves insulin sensitivity and regulates blood sugar. Low magnesium levels are associated with an increased risk of type 2 diabetes.

Sources include leafy green vegetables, nuts, seeds, whole grains, and supplements.
Recommended Intake: The RDA for adults is between 310 and 420 mg, depending on age and gender.

Chromium

Chromium is a trace mineral that improves insulin action and helps control blood sugar levels. It regulates carbohydrate and lipid metabolism, and chromium supplementation has been proven to increase glucose tolerance in diabetics.

Sources include broccoli, grape juice, potatoes, whole grains, and supplements.

Recommended Intake: The RDA for adults is 20–35 mcg; however, greater dosages may be used under medical supervision to control blood sugar levels.

Zinc

Zinc is essential for insulin synthesis and secretion in the pancreas. It also affects the shape of insulin molecules and helps insulin receptors operate properly. Zinc insufficiency can decrease insulin sensitivity and blood sugar management.

Sources include meat, seafood, beans, seeds, nuts, dairy, and supplements.

Recommended Intake: The RDA for adults is around 8–11 mg, with greater dosages available for those with deficiencies, as advised by a healthcare professional.

Alpha-lipoic acid (ALA)

Alpha-lipoic acid is an antioxidant that combats oxidative stress and inflammation, both of which are associated with insulin resistance and high blood sugar levels. ALA enhances insulin sensitivity and may help diabetics control their blood sugar levels.

Sources include spinach, broccoli, potatoes, organ meats, and supplements.
Recommended Intake: Although there is no set RDA, dosages ranging from 300 to 600 mg per day are routinely employed in studies.

B Vitamins

The B vitamins, specifically B6 (pyridoxine), B12 (cobalamin), and B7 (biotin), are involved in glucose metabolism and insulin action. These vitamins help with energy production and nerve health, which can be damaged by diabetes.

Sources include meat, eggs, dairy products, whole grains, legumes, and supplements.
Recommended Intake: RDAs for each B vitamin

vary, but typically range from 1.3–2.4 mcg for B12, 1.3–1.7 mg for B6, and 30 mcg for biotin.

Herbal Supplements for Blood Sugar

Herbal supplements have been used in traditional medicine for millennia to control blood sugar levels. Modern research confirms the effectiveness of various herbs in improving insulin sensitivity and decreasing blood sugar. Here are some important herbal supplements:

Cinnamon

Cinnamon is a famous spice renowned for its ability to reduce blood sugar levels. It contains bioactive chemicals that mimic and amplify insulin's actions, resulting in improved glucose uptake by cells.

Available forms include ground cinnamon, cinnamon extract, and capsules.

Dosage: Studies usually utilize 1-6 grams of

ground cinnamon or 250–500 mg of extract each day.

Berberine

Berberine is a chemical found in various plants, including goldenseal, barberry, and Oregon grape. It has been demonstrated to stimulate the enzyme AMP-activated protein kinase (AMPK), which regulates metabolism and blood sugar levels.

Forms include capsules and pills.
Dosage: Common doses vary from 500 to 1500 mg per day, divided into 2-3 doses.

Fenugreek

Fenugreek seeds contain soluble fiber, which slows the digestion and absorption of carbs, reducing blood sugar levels. Fenugreek also includes chemicals that may increase insulin sensitivity.

Forms include seeds, powder, and capsules.
Dosage: A typical dose is 5–50 grams of

powdered fenugreek seed or 1-2 grams of seed extract each day.

Gymnema Sylvestre.

Gymnema sylvestre is a plant used in traditional Ayurvedic therapy for diabetes. It contains chemicals that may limit sugar absorption in the intestines while increasing insulin production.

Forms include capsules and pills.
Dosage: Gymnema extract is commonly used in quantities of 200–400 mg daily.

Bitter Melon

Bitter melon, also known as bitter gourd, has chemicals with insulin-like properties that may help reduce blood sugar levels. It has been used traditionally to treat diabetes.

Forms include fresh fruit, drinks, and supplements.
Dosage: A typical dose is 50–100 mL of juice or 900–2000 mg of extract per day.

Aloe Vera

Aloe vera, known for its soothing effects, may also help with blood sugar control. It may boost insulin sensitivity and improve glycemic management in diabetics.

available in three forms: aloe vera juice, gel, and supplement.
Dosage: A typical daily dose ranges between 1 tablespoon of juice and 300–500 mg of extract.

Probiotics and Gut Health

The gut microbiome has a substantial impact on overall health, including blood sugar regulation. Probiotics, or helpful bacteria, can enhance gut health and may aid with blood sugar control.

The Gut-Glucose Connection

The gut microbiota influences metabolism, immunological function, and inflammation, all of which are involved in blood sugar management. An imbalance in gut bacteria (dysbiosis) can lead to insulin resistance and elevated blood sugar levels. Probiotics help to restore a healthy gut flora balance, which can increase insulin sensitivity and glucose metabolism.

Beneficial Probiotic Strains.

Certain probiotic strains have been investigated for their impact on blood sugar regulation. This includes:

Lactobacillus rhamnosus is known for improving gut health and maybe increasing insulin sensitivity.
Lactobacillus acidophilus may help reduce blood sugar levels and improve glycemic management.
Bifidobacterium bifidum improves overall gut health and may aid in blood sugar management.
Lactobacillus plantarum has been shown to

promote metabolic health and lower inflammatory indicators.

Sources of probiotics

1. Fermented foods include yogurt, kefir, sauerkraut, kimchi, miso, and tempeh, all of which contain probiotics.
2. Supplements: Probiotic capsules and powders can deliver high dosages of good bacteria.

Prebiotics and synbiotics

Prebiotics are nondigestible fibers that nourish beneficial gut bacteria, encouraging their proliferation and activity. Foods high in prebiotics include garlic, onions, leeks, asparagus, bananas, and whole grains.

Synbiotics combine probiotics and prebiotics to improve the survival and colonization of beneficial bacteria in the gut.

Integrating Supplements and Natural Remedies into Your Routine.

While supplements and natural therapies can help with blood sugar management, they should be used in conjunction with a balanced diet, exercise, and lifestyle modifications. Here are some suggestions for effectively using these supplements:

1. Consult a Healthcare Provider: Before beginning any supplement regimen, consult with a healthcare provider to confirm it is safe and appropriate for your unique requirements.

2. Quality Matters: To ensure potency and safety, select high-quality supplements from respected companies.

3. Begin slowly, introducing one supplement at a time, to monitor its effects and avoid potential interactions.

4. Follow Dosage Recommendations: Stick to the prescribed dosages and instructions given by the manufacturer or your healthcare provider.

5. Monitor Your Progress: Keep track of your blood sugar levels and overall health to determine how effective the supplements are.

6. Combine with Lifestyle Changes:

Supplements work best when combined with a healthy diet, frequent exercise, stress management, and proper sleep.

Chapter 8

Special Considerations.

Blood sugar regulation is an important part of health that varies greatly depending on individual circumstances, hormonal changes, and age. Understanding how to adjust blood sugar management strategies is critical to getting the best possible health outcomes. This chapter looks at managing blood sugar with diabetes, the relationship between blood sugar and hormonal health, and blood sugar management considerations for different age groups.

Managing blood sugar with diabetes

Diabetes, a chronic disorder characterized by high blood sugar levels, necessitates close monitoring to avoid complications and maintain quality of life. Lifestyle adjustments, medication, monitoring, and education are all part of an effective blood sugar control strategy.

Types of diabetes.

1. Type 1 diabetes is an autoimmune disorder in which the immune system assaults insulin-producing cells in the pancreas, resulting in little or no insulin production. It usually arises in childhood or adolescence.

2. Type 2 diabetes is characterized by insulin resistance and ultimately insulin insufficiency. It is more common in adults, although younger people are being diagnosed more frequently as obesity rates rise.

3. Gestational diabetes is a kind of diabetes that develops during pregnancy and usually resolves after childbirth. It raises the chances of having type 2 diabetes later in life.

Strategies to manage blood sugar with diabetes

1. Medication and Insulin Therapy

Type 1 diabetes: The body cannot manufacture

insulin; hence, insulin therapy is required. Various types of insulin (fast, short, intermediate, and long-acting) are used to control blood sugar levels throughout the day.

Type 2 diabetes can be managed with oral drugs (such as metformin, sulfonylureas, or DPP-4 inhibitors), injectable medications (GLP-1 receptor agonists), and, if necessary, insulin therapy.

2. Blood Sugar Monitoring

Self-monitoring: Regular blood sugar testing with a glucometer allows people to understand how food, exercise, and medication affect their blood sugar levels.

Continuous Glucose Monitoring (CGM): CGM systems give real-time blood sugar levels throughout the day, allowing you to discover patterns and make informed management decisions.

3. Dietary Management

Carbohydrate Counting: Monitoring carbohydrate intake can help prevent blood sugar rises. Understanding how various foods affect blood sugar is critical.

Balanced Diet: Eating whole grains, lean proteins, healthy fats, and plenty of veggies helps to regulate blood sugar levels.

Glycemic Index (GI): Eating low-GI meals, which digest more slowly, can help reduce sudden blood sugar rises.

4. Exercise

Regular physical activity increases insulin sensitivity and lowers blood sugar levels. Resistance training, as well as cardiovascular exercises (such as walking, jogging, and swimming), are useful.

Blood sugar levels should be monitored before and after exercise to avoid hypoglycemia.

5. Education and Support

Diabetes education programs offer helpful information on managing the condition, such as lifestyle changes, medication adherence, and coping strategies.

Support groups and therapy can help with the emotional and psychological aspects of living with diabetes.

Blood sugar and hormone health

Hormones play an important function in controlling blood sugar. Understanding the relationship between blood sugar and hormonal health is critical for effective management, particularly in diabetes and metabolic syndrome.

Insulin

The pancreas produces insulin, which is the major hormone responsible for reducing blood sugar levels. It promotes the absorption of glucose into cells for energy or storage. Insulin resistance, in which cells become less receptive to insulin, is a hallmark of type 2 diabetes.

Glucagon

Glucagon, another pancreatic hormone, functions in the opposite way that insulin does, elevating blood sugar levels. When blood sugar levels fall below normal, it signals the liver to release stored glucose into the bloodstream. A balance between insulin and glucagon is required to maintain stable blood sugar levels.

Cortisol

The adrenal glands create cortisol, which is known as the stress hormone. It raises blood sugar by increasing gluconeogenesis (the creation of glucose from non-carbohydrate sources) in the liver. Chronic stress and raised cortisol levels can cause insulin resistance and high blood sugar levels.

Thyroid hormones

Thyroid hormones (T3 and T4) control metabolism, which includes how carbs are processed. Hypothyroidism (low thyroid function) can slow metabolism, resulting in weight gain and insulin resistance, whereas hyperthyroidism (overactive thyroid) can accelerate metabolism and occasionally cause hypoglycemia.

Estrogen and progesterone.

Women's estrogen and progesterone levels fluctuate during the menstrual cycle, pregnancy, and menopause, altering blood sugar levels.

Estrogen normally enhances insulin sensitivity, but progesterone can offset this effect, resulting in higher blood sugar levels during the luteal phase of the menstrual cycle.

Menstrual period: Blood sugar levels can change throughout the period, with some women having higher levels during the luteal phase (after ovulation) due to elevated progesterone.

Pregnancy: Pregnancy hormones can promote insulin resistance, resulting in gestational diabetes. Careful monitoring and treatment are required to ensure the health of both the mother and the infant.

Menopause: Hormonal changes during menopause can impair blood sugar regulation. Postmenopausal women may have increased insulin resistance and are more likely to acquire type 2 diabetes.

Blood sugar management for different age groups.

Blood sugar management solutions should be adapted to each age group's specific physiological and lifestyle requirements. This section discusses blood sugar management for children, adults, and older persons.

Children and adolescents

Managing blood sugar in children and adolescents with diabetes or at risk of getting it necessitates unique measures to promote their growth and development.

1. Education and Empowerment
Educating children and their families about diabetes management is critical, including good food, exercise, and blood sugar monitoring.
Encouraging youngsters to take an active role in their own care promotes lifetime health practices.

2. School and Social Activities:
Coordinating with school administrators and activity leaders is necessary to ensure that children manage their diabetes at school and during extracurricular activities.
Planning for special occasions, such as parties and sporting events, can help keep blood sugar levels consistent.

3. Psychosocial support.
Addressing the emotional and social issues associated with diabetes is critical for children and adolescents. Support groups and counseling might help individuals deal with the stress and worry associated with their disease.

4. Growth and Development.
Monitoring growth and development is critical, as diabetes care requirements may vary during puberty. Regular visits to a healthcare provider help ensure that blood sugar control promotes healthy growth.

Adults

For adults, regulating blood sugar entails combining work, family commitments, and lifestyle modifications to avoid or manage diabetes.

1. Work-life balance.
Fitting good food and regular exercise into a hectic work schedule necessitates preparation and commitment. Meal planning and making time for physical activity can assist.
Stress management practices, such as mindfulness and relaxation exercises, are essential for blood sugar regulation.

2. Preventive Health
Regular health screenings, including blood sugar tests and monitoring for consequences like cardiovascular disease, are critical for early detection and treatment.
Maintaining a healthy weight through diet and exercise improves insulin sensitivity and prevents type 2 diabetes.

3. Family Support

Involving family members in diabetes treatment creates a supportive environment. Family activities that encourage healthy eating and activity benefit everyone.

Educating family members about diabetes allows them to grasp the condition and provide appropriate assistance.

Older Adults

Older people may experience specific blood sugar management issues due to age-related changes in metabolism, mobility, and comorbidities.

1. Simplified management plans.

Simplifying diabetes management programs, such as medication regimens and monitoring routines, can help older people stick to their treatment.

Using pill organizers and reminders can help with medication adherence.

2. Nutritional Needs

It is critical to provide enough nutrition for older people because their dietary needs and tastes may differ. Nutrient-dense diets and balanced meals help to keep blood sugar levels constant. Addressing oral problems and swallowing difficulties can boost meal intake and nutrition.

3. Physical activity.

Adapting exercise regimens to accommodate mobility restrictions and other health issues assists older people in remaining active. Low-impact activities such as walking, swimming, and chair workouts are advantageous.

Regular physical activity promotes muscle mass retention, insulin sensitivity, and overall well-being.

4. Monitoring and Complications

Regular blood sugar monitoring and routine health screenings aid in the detection and management of problems like neuropathy, retinopathy, and cardiovascular disease.

Coordinating care among many healthcare

providers ensures that diabetes and other health disorders are managed comprehensively.

Adding Special Considerations to Blood Sugar Management

To effectively manage blood sugar, a personalized approach is required that takes into account specific health conditions, hormonal changes, and age-related needs. Here are some ways to incorporate these special factors into a complete blood sugar management plan:

1. Personalized Care Plans
Collaborate with healthcare practitioners to create tailored treatment plans that reflect patients' unique requirements, preferences, and health goals.
Review and amend care plans on a regular basis, taking into account changes in health status, lifestyle, and treatment response.

2. Education and awareness.
Stay current on the latest research and developments in diabetes treatment, hormonal

health, and age-related health issues.

Participate in educational programs and support groups to improve your knowledge and abilities in blood sugar management.

3. Holistic Approach

Take a comprehensive approach to health that includes food, exercise, stress management, and proper sleep hygiene. Consider using complementary therapies and natural remedies as part of a comprehensive approach.

Focus on mental and emotional well-being, acknowledging the impact of stress and psychological

Factors affecting blood sugar regulation.

4. Proactive monitoring

Monitor blood sugar levels on a regular basis and preserve extensive records to spot patterns and make informed management decisions.

Track and analyze blood sugar levels using technology such as continuous glucose monitoring and health apps.

5. Support Systems

Create a solid support system that includes family, friends, healthcare providers, and peer groups.

Encourage open communication with support systems about blood sugar management issues and triumphs.

Managing blood sugar successfully necessitates a thorough awareness of a variety of aspects, including diabetes, hormonal health, and age-related concerns. Individuals can improve their entire health and well-being by following personalized techniques and being educated. This complete approach ensures that specific considerations are built into regular activities, allowing individuals to take control of their health and confidently negotiate the difficulties of blood sugar management.

Chapter 9

Creating Your Personal Blood Sugar Plan

Blood sugar management involves a specialized approach that takes into account individual needs, goals, and circumstances. A personalized blood sugar plan can help you gain control of your glucose levels, improve your general health, and avoid issues. This chapter will walk you through the process of creating objectives, tracking progress, forming a support network, and overcoming obstacles on your path to balanced blood sugar.

Setting goals and tracking progress

Setting specific, attainable goals and monitoring your progress are critical elements in developing a successful blood sugar management strategy.

Goals provide guidance and inspiration, whereas tracking allows you to stay on track and make the required changes.

Establishing SMART goals

SMART goals are specific, measurable, achievable, relevant, and time-bound. This framework guarantees that your goals are clear and attainable, increasing your chances of success.

1. Specific
Define your goals clearly. Instead of saying, "I want to lower my blood sugar," define what you hope to achieve, such as "I want to lower my fasting blood sugar levels to between 80 and 120 mg/dL."

2. Measurable
Include criteria for measuring progress. For instance, "I will check my blood sugar levels every morning before breakfast and log the results."

3. Achievable

Set realistic, attainable goals. For example, "I will incorporate a 30-minute walk into my daily routine."

4. Relevant

Make sure your goals are related to your entire health and wellness. For instance, "I will reduce my intake of sugary snacks to manage my blood sugar levels better."

5. Time-bound

Determine a timeframe for reaching your objectives. For example, "I will achieve my target blood sugar levels within three months."

Short- and long-term goals

Balancing short-term and long-term goals helps you stay motivated and gives you a clear path for your trip.

Short-Term Goals

Prioritize immediate improvements and behaviors that can be introduced quickly. For instance, "I will eat a balanced breakfast every day this week" and "I will walk for 30 minutes, five days a week."

long-term goals.
Aim for long-term improvements in blood sugar control. For instance, "I will lower my HbA1c level to below 6.5% within six months" and "I will maintain a healthy weight through balanced nutrition and regular exercise."

Tracking Progress

Regularly tracking your progress allows you to remain accountable and make informed changes to your plan.

1. Blood sugar monitoring
Use a glucometer to monitor your blood sugar levels regularly. Keep a journal of your readings, noting the time of day, what you ate, and any physical activity.
Consider adopting a continuous glucose monitor (CGM) for real-time data on your blood sugar levels and trends.

2. Diet and Exercise Logs

Record your daily food intake, including portion sizes and carbohydrate content. Tracking your food helps you detect patterns and make the required changes.

Keep track of your physical activity, including the type, duration, and intensity of each workout. This helps you assess the effect of exercise on your blood sugar levels.

3. Health metrics

Monitor other health indicators like weight, blood pressure, and cholesterol levels. These indicators offer a complete picture of your overall health and progress.

4. Goal Review

Regularly examine your goals and progress. Assess what is working and what isn't, and make the required revisions to your plan.

Building a Support System

A solid support system is essential for effectively managing blood sugar levels. Support from family, friends, healthcare providers, and peer groups can offer motivation, accountability, and practical support.

Family and friends.

1. Educate your support network.
Educate your family and friends on blood sugar management and your individual requirements. Understanding your goals and obstacles enables them to deliver greater support.

2. Involve them in your journey.
Involve your loved ones in your health journey. Invite them to join you in healthy activities, such as making nutritious meals or exercising together.
Communicate your progress and difficulties to them. Open communication promotes a helpful and understanding workplace.

3. Set boundaries and expectations.

Set clear boundaries and expectations for your requirements and preferences. For example, urge that they avoid bringing enticing sugary treats into the house.

Healthcare providers

1. Regular check-ups

Make regular appointments with your healthcare providers to monitor your progress, change your treatment plan, and discuss any concerns.

Talk about your objectives and challenges with your doctor, dietician, and diabetes educator. They can offer helpful advice and support.

2. Access to resources

Use the resources supplied by your healthcare team, such as educational materials, diet plans, and exercise advice.

Consider joining diabetes management classes or workshops offered by your healthcare practitioner.

Peer support groups

1. Join support groups.
Join a local or online support group for people who are managing their blood sugar or living with diabetes. Connecting with individuals who have had similar experiences can offer encouragement and emotional support.
Take part in group conversations, share your experiences, and learn from others' accomplishments and struggles.

2. Find a buddy system.
Form a partnership with a buddy or other support group member to ensure mutual accountability. A buddy system might help you stay motivated and focused on your goals.

Overcoming Challenges

Managing blood sugar levels is not easy. Identifying possible hurdles and devising solutions to overcome them is critical to long-term success.

Common Challenges and Solutions.

1. Dietary temptations
Challenge: Cravings for sugary or high-carb foods can disrupt your blood sugar management strategy.
Solution: Keep nutritious snacks on hand, plan your meals, and practice mindful eating to reduce urges. Allow yourself a few treats in moderation to avoid feeling deprived.

2. Inconsistent Routine
Challenge: A hectic or irregular schedule might make it challenging to keep a consistent routine for meals, exercise, and blood sugar monitoring.
Solution: Plan and prepare meals in advance, schedule exercise sessions, and create reminders for blood sugar tests. Flexibility and adaptability are crucial.

3. Emotional and mental health.
Difficulty: Stress, worry, and sadness can affect blood sugar levels and impede self-care

attempts.

Solution: Use stress-relieving techniques like meditation, yoga, or deep breathing exercises. Seek professional help from a counselor or therapist if necessary.

4. Social situations

Difficulty: Food and beverages on social occasions can interfere with your blood sugar regulation.

Solution: Plan ahead by eating a nutritious snack before the event, choosing healthier options, and managing portion amounts. Don't be afraid to explain your dietary requirements to hosts.

5. Plateaus and Setbacks

Challenge: Reaching a plateau or suffering setbacks can be frustrating and reduce motivation.

Solution: Reevaluate your goals and strategies, seek help from your healthcare practitioner, and celebrate minor accomplishments. Remember that progress is not always linear.

Building Resilience

1. Positive mindset
Cultivate a positive mindset by focusing on your achievements and progress. To keep yourself motivated and resilient, practice thankfulness and self-compassion.

2. Problem-solving skills
Improve your problem-solving abilities so you can deal with issues as they arise. Break down challenges into smaller, more manageable steps and consider alternative solutions.

3. Adaptability
Take a flexible and responsive approach. Recognize that plans may need to be changed and that setbacks are a normal part of the process.

4. Self-Care
Prioritize self-care by getting adequate sleep, staying hydrated, and engaging in things that offer you joy and relaxation.

Creating a Comprehensive Blood Sugar Management Plan

Integrating these factors into a complete blood sugar management plan takes careful planning and constant modifications. Here is a step-by-step approach to building your personalized plan:

1. Assessment and Goal Setting
Conduct a full evaluation of your present health, lifestyle, and blood sugar levels.
Set SMART blood sugar control goals that take into account both immediate and long-term objectives.

2. Developing Action Plans
Develop thorough strategies for diet, exercise, medicine, and monitoring. Specify the steps you will take to achieve your objectives.

3. Implementing Support Systems
Identify and engage your support systems, including family, friends, healthcare providers, and peer groups.

Schedule regular check-ins with your support network to ensure accountability and encouragement.

4. Tracking and Monitoring

Use tools like blood sugar logs, diet and exercise journals, and health apps to track your progress. Regularly evaluate your data to find trends, accomplishments, and places for development.

5. Review and Adjustments

Set up regular reviews of your strategy with your healthcare provider. Make the required changes based on your progress and any additional problems.

Stay up-to-date on new research, medications, and blood sugar management practices.

6. Maintaining motivation

Celebrate your victories, no matter how minor, and use them as an incentive to keep going.

Maintain contact with your support network and seek assistance when experiencing obstacles.

Developing a personalized blood sugar strategy is a dynamic process that entails defining specific goals, establishing a strong support network, and conquering obstacles with perseverance and adaptation. By following the procedures provided in this chapter, you may design a thorough strategy tailored to your individual requirements and circumstances. Remember that managing blood sugar is a journey that involves constant effort and dedication, but with the correct strategy and assistance, you may achieve better control and enhance your overall health and well-being.

Chapter 10

Success Story and Testimonials

Hearing from individuals who have successfully overcome similar issues can be extremely inspiring and motivating on the path to regulating blood sugar levels and overall health. This chapter collects real-life stories, lessons learnedlearned, and practical advice from people who have improved their health throughthrough careful blood sugar management. These success stories demonstrate the value of endurance, the significance of individualized solutions, and the influence of supportive networks.

Real-Life Experiences

Emily's Transformation: From Diagnosis toto Mastery

Emily was diagnosed with type 2 diabetes at the age of 45. At the time, she lived a sedentary lifestyle, ate a lot of sugary snacks, and knew little about diabetes. The diagnosis was a wake-up call that drove her to change her lifestyle.

1. Initial Struggles and Breakthroughs

Emily experienced initial challenges, such as comprehending her condition and making nutritional changes. She recalls being overwhelmed by the volume of information and lifestyle modifications required.

Emily's breakthrough occurred when she attended a diabetic education session. The program equipped her with the knowledge and resources she required to effectively manage her disease. She learnedlearned about carbohydrate counting, the benefits of physical activity, and how to keep track of her blood sugar levels.

2. Building a Support System

Emily established a strong support network that included her family, friends, and the healthcare staff. Her husband joined her in embracing a healthy lifestyle, making the trip less isolated and more joyful.

She also joined a local diabetes support group, where she met otherssuffering from suffering from similar issues. Sharing experiences and tips with peers gave both emotional support and practical help.

3. Adopting a New Lifestyle

Emily began incorporating regular exercise into her routine. She started with daily walks and then added strength training and yoga. Exercise not only helped her manage her blood sugar levels, but it also boosted her attitude and vitality.

She changed her diet by focusing on natural foods, limiting refined sugars, and adopting portion control. Meal preparation and planning became crucial components of her routine, making it easier to adhere to her nutritional goals.

4. Sustained Success

Emily's blood sugar levels eventually regulated, and she lost significant weight. Her HbA1c values decreaseddecreased from 8.5% to 6.2%, demonstrating her commitment and hard work.

Emily highlights the value of constancy and patience. She understands that setbacks are inevitable, but she sees them as opportunities to learn and modify.

John's journey: embracing a holistic approach.

John, a 55-year-old businessman, was diagnosed with prediabetes following a routine examination. Concerned about his health and the danger of developing type 2 diabetes, John made the decision to act immediately.

1. Awareness and Education

John dedicated himself to understanding blood sugar regulation. He researched books, attended workshops, and spoke with his doctor to better understand the consequences of prediabetes and the procedures necessary to reverse it.

His studies prompted him to take a comprehensive approach that includes dietary adjustments, frequent exercise, stress management, and mindfulness activities.

2. Dietary Changes

John adopted a plant-based diet high in vegetables, fruits, healthy grains, and lean proteins. He cut back on processed foods and sugars, opting for more nutrient-dense options.

He became more aware of portion sizes and meal time, providing a balanced diet throughout the day to avoid blood sugar spikes.

3. Incorporating Physical Activity

Despite his busy schedule, John prioritized physical activity. He added 30 minutes of exercise to his daily routine, which included a variety of cardiovascular workouts, weight training, and flexibility exercises.

He discovered that regular exercise not only helped him control his blood sugar levels but also gave him more energy and lowered his stress.

4. Stress management and mindfulness

Recognizing the effects of stress on blood sugar levels, John integrated stress management practices into his daily routine. He employed meditation, deep breathing exercises, and awareness to keep calm and focused.

He also prioritized sleep, acknowledging its importance toto overall health and blood sugar management.

5. Results and Reflections

Within six months, John's prediabetes was resolved, and his blood sugar levels returned to normal. His holistic approach resulted in improved health markers, such as lower cholesterol and blood pressure.

John describes his journey as a transforming event. He highlights the value of a proactive approach as well as the advantages of a comprehensive, long-term lifestyle adjustment.

Sarah's Story: Managing Blood Sugar withwith PCOS

Sarah, a 30-year-old woman, was diagnosed with PCOS and suffered from insulin resistance. Managing her blood sugar levels became critical for relieving her symptoms and enhancing her general health.

1. Understanding thet condition

Sarah's PCOS diagnosis came with a slew of complications, including irregular menstrual periods, weight gain, and high blood sugar levels. Her healthcare practitioner discussed the link between insulin resistance and PCOS, emphasizing the importance of blood sugar control.

She researched PCOS and insulin resistance, participating in online forums and attending seminars to better understand the issue.

2. Tailored Dietary Approach

Sarah collaborated with a dietitian to create a meal plan that addressed her insulin resistance and promoted hormonal wellness. She followed a low-glycemic index (GI) diet that consisted primarily of whole grains, lean meats, and healthy fats.

She used fiber-rich diets to delay sugar absorption and increase insulin sensitivity. Sarah also practiced mindful eating, paying attention to her body's hunger and satiety signals.

3.   Exercise   and   physicalphysical activityactivity

Regular exercise became an essential component of Sarah's management strategy. She practiced aerobics, strength training, and yoga.

Exercise helped to control her blood sugar, reduce stress, and enhance her mood. Sarah discovered that consistency was crucial, so she made exercise a non-negotiable element of her regimen.

4. Hormone Balance and Stress Reduction

Sarah experimented with several techniques to naturally balance her hormones. She used supplements such as inositol, which is known to increase insulin sensitivity in women with PCOS.

Stress management was critical, as it could aggravate her symptoms. Sarah used yoga, meditation, and journaling to reduce stress and improve relaxation.

5. Achieving Balance

Sarah's blood sugar levels gradually regulated, and her PCOS symptoms improved. Her menstrual periods became regular, and she gained a healthy weight.

Sarah's story emphasizes the significance of a multifaceted approach to blood sugar management in the context of hormonal health. She advises those with PCOS to educate themselves, seek professional help, and stay focused on their health goals.

Lessons Learned and Success Strategies

The success stories mentioned above provide vital insights and practical advice for anybody seeking to manage blood sugar levels. Here are some major findings and actionable ideas that emerged from these experiences:

Education and awarenessawareness.

1. Learn about your condition.
Understanding your health issue is the first step toward successful management. Educate yourself on blood sugar regulation, the effects of various diets, and the function of exercise.
Use resources,resources, including books,the internet, the internet, workshops, and discussions with healthcare providers,providers, to broaden your understanding.

2. Stay informed.
Stay current on the latest research and advances in blood sugar management. Continuous learning allows you to modify and refine your techniques based on fresh facts.

Personalized Plans

1. Set realistic goals.
Establish specific, measurable, attainable, relevant, and time-bound goals (SMART). Break

down huge goals into smaller, more doable steps to stay motivated and track progress.

Approach your goals with patience and flexibility. Adjust them as needed to reflect your success and any new challenges that occur.

2. Tailor youryour approachapproach.

Tailor your plan to your own lifestyle, interests, and health needs. What works for one person may not work for another, so identify the tactics that are most effective for you.

When creating your food, exercise, and stress management routines, take into account your work schedule, family commitments, and personal preferences.

Building a Support System

1. Engage youryour networknetwork.

Involve your family and friends in your healthcare journey. Share your goals and progress with them, and ask for their support and encouragement.

Participate in support groups, both online and offline, to connect with people facing similar issues. Sharing experiences and recommendations with peers can provide useful information and motivation.

2. Professional Guidance
Collaborate with healthcare professionals, such as doctors, dietitians, and diabetes educators, to create and refine your blood sugar management strategy.
Regular check-ups and discussions help to monitor your progress and address any issues or modifications that may be required.

Overcoming Challenges

1. Identify and address obstacles.
Anticipate future obstacles and devise solutions to overcome them. Dietary temptations, unpredictable routines, and emotional stress are all common difficulties.
Plan ahead of time by eating well, exercising on a regular basis, and practicing stress-management skills.

2. Stay resilientresilient.

Develop a positive outlook and maintain resilience in the face of setbacks. Instead of viewing problems as failures, consider them chances to learn and improve.

Recognize minor accomplishments and improvements along the way. Recognize your accomplishments and use them as inspiration to continue your efforts.

Holistic Health Approach.

1. Comprehensive Lifestyle Changes

A comprehensive approach that includes nutrition, exercise, stress management, and proper sleep is essential for long-term success. Prioritize a healthy and sustainable lifestyle above fast cures or drastic tactics.

2. Mindfulness and selfself-care

Practice mindfulness and self-care to sustain mental and emotional health. Meditation, deep breathing exercises, and journaling

Aling can help you manage stress and relax.
Get enough sleep, as poor sleep can harm blood sugar levels and overall health.

Success stories about people who have successfully regulated their blood sugar levels using tailored tactics, supportive networks, and holistic approaches serve as strong reminders of what is possible. These real-life experiences and lessons acquired provide useful advice and motivation for anyone embarking on a similar path. You can attain balanced blood sugar levels and better general well-being by educating yourself, setting realistic goals, forming a strong support system, facing problems with fortitude, and taking a complete approach to healthcare.

Chapter 11

The Future of Blood Sugar Management.

When we consider the future of blood sugar management, we see a quickly changing landscape characterized by novel technologies, pioneering rescarch, and a better understanding of metabolic health. The combination of digital health, customized medicine, and scientific research promises to revolutionize how we monitor, treat, and manage blood sugar levels. This chapter delves into the most recent advances in blood sugar monitoring and treatment, the role of technology, and future research approaches that have the potential to transform the field.

Innovations in Monitoring and Treatment

Continuous glucose monitoring (CGM).

Continuous Glucose Monitoring (CGM) technologies have transformed blood sugar management by delivering real-time glucose values throughout the day and night. These devices use a tiny sensor implanted under the skin to assess interstitial glucose levels, which has various advantages over standard fingerstick approaches.

1. Real-time monitoringmonitoring
Continuous glucose monitoring (CGM) systems provide real-time input on blood glucose levels, allowing users to identify trends and patterns that might otherwise be overlooked with periodic fingerstick testing.
Alerts and alarms can inform users of imminent hypoglycemia or hyperglycemia, allowing for prompt interventions.

2. Data--Driven Insights

The extensive data offered by CGMs may be examined to detect triggers and trends, allowing users and healthcare practitioners to make more informed food, exercise, and medication decisions.

Integration with smartphone apps and cloud platforms enables easy data tracking and sharing with healthcare experts, resulting in more tailored and proactive care.

3. Advances in Sensor Technology

Recent advances in sensor technology have resulted in smaller, more comfortable, and longerlonger-lasting CGM sensors. Newer devices require fewer calibrations and provide better accuracy.

Future advancements seek to create entirely non-invasive CGM systems that do not require sensor insertion, hence increasing user convenience and compliance.

Artificial pancreaticpancreatic systems

Artificial pancreas devices, often known as closed-loop insulin administration systems, are a significant advancement in diabetes management. These systems use CGM technologies, insulin pumps, and advanced algorithms to automate insulin delivery.

1. Automated Insulin Delivery
The artificial pancreas continuously analyzes blood glucose levels and changes insulin delivery in real time to imitate the operation of a healthy pancreas.
This automation alleviates the stress of manual insulin dosing, promotes more stable blood glucose levels, and reduces the danger of hypoglycemia and hyperglycemia.

2. Improved Quality of Life
Users of artificial pancreas systems claima higher a higher quality of life since the technology eliminates the need for continuous

monitoring and decision-making.

Better glycemic control achieved through these systems can result in fewer diabetic complications and better long-term health outcomes.

3. Future Directions

Current research is aimed at improving the algorithms used in artificial pancreas systems to account for aspects like meal composition, physical activity, and stress.

Research is also underway to develop dual-hormone systems that supply both insulin and glucagon, allowing for even more precise control of blood glucose levels.

Novel medications and therapies

The creation of new drugs and therapies is another interesting area in blood sugar management. Pharmaceutical and biotechnology advances are resulting in more effective and focused treatments.

1. GLP-1 receptor agonists

Glucagon-like peptide-1 (GLP-1) receptor agonists are a type of drug that stimulates insulin production, inhibits glucagon release, and slows gastric emptying, resulting in better blood glucose management.

These drugs also encourage weight loss, which is beneficial to many people with type 2 diabetes.

2. SGLT2 inhibitors

SGLT2 inhibitors impede glucose reabsorption in the kidneys, resulting in increased glucose excretion in the urine.

This method lowers blood glucose levels and has been demonstrated to improve cardiovascular and renal health.

3. Gene-Gene- and cell-basedcell-based therapiestherapies

Gene therapy and stem cell studies show promise for healing diabetes. Efforts are underway to discover medicines that can regrow insulin-producing beta cells or fix genetic abnormalities that cause diabetes.

Encapsulation techniques are intended to shield transplanted beta cells from immunological attack, perhaps providing a long-term treatment for type 1 diabetes.

The role of technology

Digital healthhealth platformsplatforms

Blood sugar management is being transformed by digital health platforms, which combine numerous tools and resources into integrated, user-friendly ecosystems.

1.Comprehensive healthhealth managementt.
Digital systems provide comprehensive health management solutions, including CGM data, diet and exercise tracking, medication administration, and more.
With one easy-to-use interface, users can establish goals, receive personalized advice, and track their progress.

2. Telemedicine andand Remote Monitoring

Telemedicine enables virtual consultations with healthcare providers, making it easier for people to get timely care and support without having to visit a clinic.

Remote monitoring systems enable healthcare providers to track patients' blood sugar levels and other health data in real time, allowing for more preemptive interventions and individualized care regimens.

3. AI and machinemachine learninglearning

Artificial intelligence (AI) and machine learning (ML) systems can scan massive datasets to detect patterns and forecast blood glucose levels. These technologies can provideprovide consumers with individualized insights and recommendations, allowing them to make more educated health decisions.

Mobile applications and wearables

Mobile apps and wearable devices are quickly becoming essential tools for blood sugar management, providing convenience, motivation, and data-driven insights.

1. Mobile Apps for Diabetes Management
Diabetes management applications include blood sugar reporting, food planning, carb counting, and exercise tracking.
Many apps work seamlessly with CGM and insulin pump systems, giving users more exact control over blood glucose levels.

2. Wearable fitnessfitness trackerstrackers.
Wearable fitness trackers track physical activity, heart rate, sleep habits, and other parameters. These devices collect useful data that can be utilized to better understand how lifestyle factors affect blood sugar levels.
Integration with health applications enables users to link physical activity to blood glucose trends, allowing them to tailor their exercise regimens for improved glucose control.

3. Smart Insulin Pens and Patches
Smart insulin pens and patches are connected with sensors and Bluetooth connectivity,

allowing for automatic logging of insulin doses and timing.

These devices can notify users of missed doses, provide dosage reminders, and interact with mobile apps for comprehensive diabetes care.

Gamification and behavior change

Gamification and behavioral change strategies are being used to improve user engagement and compliance with blood sugar management plans.

1. Gamified Health Apps
Gamified health apps incorporate game design features like points, badges, and leaderboards to encourage users to follow their diabetes control goals.
These apps can make blood glucose monitoring, good eating, and exercise more pleasurable and rewarding.

2. Behavioral Change Programs
Digital health platforms frequently include behavioral change programs that encourage healthy behaviors through approaches such as

goal setting, self-monitoring, feedback, and social support.

Users can benefit from personalized coaching and support in developing and maintaining long-term habits that improve blood glucose control.

Future research directions

Precision Medicine

Precision medicine tries to personalize therapies to each patient's unique traits, taking into account genetics, environment, and lifestyle.

1. Genomic insights

Genomic research is shedding light on the hereditary factors that contribute to diabetes and individual treatment outcomes. This information may lead to more tailored and effective therapies.

Genetic testing can helphelp identify those who are at risk of developing diabetes, allowing for early intervention and individualized preventative efforts.

2. Personalized Treatment Plans
Precision medicine approaches can create individualized treatment regimens based on a person's specific profile. This includes selecting the most effective drugs, making food recommendations, and following an exercise plan.
Advances in biotechnology may enable the development of personalized biologics and gene therapies based on an individual's genetic composition.

Microbiome Research

The human gut microbiome is important for metabolic health, and research is being conducted to better understand its impact on blood glucose regulation.

1. The Microbiome and Diabetes Connection
Research indicates that the composition and diversity of the gut microbiome can affect

insulin sensitivity, inflammation, and glucose metabolism.

Researchers are looking into how changes to the microbiome, such as probiotics, prebiotics, and dietary interventions, can enhance blood glucose control.

2. Targeted microbiome therapies

Future therapeutics may entail targeted manipulation of the gut microbiome to boost good bacterial strains while inhibiting toxic ones.

Personalized microbiome treatments could be created based on an individual's microbial profile, improving theirtheir effect on blood glucose management.

AI and Big Data

AI and big data are revolutionizing healthcare research by providingproviding strong tools for analyzing large datasets and discovering new insights.

1. Predictive analytics

AI systems can evaluate massive datasets to forecast blood glucose trends, detect risk factors, and suggest personalized interventions.

Predictive analytics can helphelp healthcare providers anticipate and prevent issues, resulting in better patient outcomes.

2. Drug Discovery and Development.

Artificial intelligence is being used to speed up drug discovery and development by identifying possible therapeutic targets and forecasting the efficacy of novel molecules.

Machine learning algorithms can use clinical trial data and real-world information to improve treatment protocols and discover the most effective medicines.

Telemedicine and Remote Care

Telemedicine and remote care are increasing access to diabetes treatment services, especially among impoverished populations.

1. Improving Access to Care

Telemedicine can help bridge healthcare access gaps by offering remote consultations and support to people living in rural or underserved locations.

Remote monitoring systems provide for continuous care and assistance, decreasing the need for frequent in-person visits while enhancing patient outcomes.

2. Integrating Remote Monitoring and Clinical Care

Integrating remote monitoring data into clinical treatment enables more proactive and tailored management.

of blood glucose levels.

Real-time data enables healthcare providers to make informed judgments, change treatment plans, and give prompt treatments.

Technological improvements, innovative treatments, and revolutionary research are all poised to change blood sugar management in thenext few next few years. Continuous glucose monitoring, artificial pancreas devices, and new drugs are already making substantial advances in blood glucose management. The combination of digital health platforms, smartphone apps, and wearable devices provides unparalleled ease and data-driven insights. Precision medicine, microbiome research, and AI-powered predictive analytics present the potential of personalized and successful therapies based on individual needs.

As these advances progress, they will enable people to take control of their health, improve their quality of life, and lessen the impact of diabetes and other blood sugar-related illnesses. The future is bright, and the opportunities are limitless as we transition to a more connected, personalized, and proactive approach to blood sugar management.

Conclusion

Recap of Key Points

Throughout this book, we have looked at the key parts of blood sugar regulation, emphasizing the need toto maintainmaintain stable blood sugar levels for overall health and well-being. Here's a summary of the important themes discussed:

1. Understanding Blood Sugar's Impact:
Blood sugar (glucose) is the body's major source of energy. Maintaining stable blood sugar levels is critical for avoiding chronic illnesses such as diabetes and cardiovascular disease.
The glycemic index (GI) and glycemic load (GL) of foods can affect blood sugar levels. Choosing low-GI and low-GL foods contributes to stable blood sugar levels.

2. Dietary Influences on Blood Sugar Control:
Controlling blood sugar requires a well-balanced diet rich in whole grains, lean proteins, healthy fats, and fiber. Avoiding processed foods and

refined sugars can help prevent blood sugar increases.

Meal planning and mindful eating have a substantial impact on blood sugar levels. Regular meals and snacks help you stay energized and avoid overeating.

3. Exercise and Blood Sugar Management:
Regular physical activity increases insulin sensitivity and lowers blood sugar levels. Both aerobic and strength training are useful.

Including activity in regular activities, such as ascending the stairs or walking after meals, helps improve blood sugar control.

4. Lifestyle Changes for Blood Sugar Management:
Stress reduction strategies such as mindfulness, meditation, and deep breathing exercises are essential for blood sugar regulation.

Proper sleep is critical for overall health and blood sugar regulation. Aim for 7-9 hours of restful sleep each night.

Reducing exposure to environmental contaminants, such as endocrine disruptors, can help with hormonal balance and blood sugar management.

5. Supplements and natural remedies:
Essential vitamins and minerals,minerals, including magnesium, chromium, and vitamin D,D, help regulate blood sugar levels.
Herbal supplements such as berberine, cinnamon, and fenugreek can help regulate blood sugar levels.
Probiotics and gut health have been related to better blood sugar control and overall metabolic health.

6. Special Considerations:
Managing blood sugar with diabetes necessitates a combination of medication, lifestyle adjustments, and frequent monitoring.
Hormonal health, including thyroid, cortisol, and reproductive hormones, might affect blood sugar levels.
Blood sugar management measures should be age-appropriate, taking into account the specific needs of children, adults, and the elderly.

7. Creating Your Personal Blood Sugar Plan:
Setting SMART objectives and measuring progress helps you stay motivated and focused on your blood sugar management journey.

Creating a solid support network of family, friends, healthcare providers, and peer groups provides both encouragement and accountability. Overcoming problems with tenacity and adaptability leads to long-term success in blood sugar management.

Encouragement on Your Journey

Starting the road to managing your blood sugar levels is an important step toward better health and well-being. To make long-term lifestyle changes, you must be dedicated, patient, and willing. Remember, you are not alone on this path. There is support accessible, and resources are abundant to help you attain your objectives.

1. Stay committed:
Consistency is essential. Small, regular efforts might provide huge results over time. Celebrate

your accomplishments and remain focused on your long-term health objectives.

2. Seek support:
Don't be afraid to seek help from healthcare professionals, family, friends, and support groups. Sharing your experiences and problems can bring helpful insights and encouragement.

3. Be kind to yourself.
Understand that setbacks are a normal part of any endeavor. Be nice to yourself and see obstacles as chances to learn and grow. Your perseverance and resilience will result in success.

4. Stay informed:
Continue to learn about new studies, tactics, and tools for blood sugar management. Staying informed allows you to make the best choices for your health.

5. Enjoy the journey:
Enjoy the process of maintaining your health. Experiment with new dishes, engage in varied

physical activities, and reap the benefits of a healthier lifestyle.

Final Thoughts

Managing blood sugar levels requires a diverse approach that includes nutrition, exercise, lifestyle modifications, and emotional well-being. Understanding the science of blood sugar regulation and using practical techniques will help you take control of your health and avoid the chronic problems associated with high blood sugar.

This book provides a thorough approach to blood sugar management, including insights, recommendations, and encouragement to help you on your way to better health. Remember that each person's experience is unique, and what works for one may not work for another. Maintain your flexibility, patience, and trust in the process.

Your dedication to managing your blood sugar levels will not only improve your quality of life but will also benefit your long-term health and well-being. Embrace this path with an open heart and a good attitude, and you will reap the benefits of a healthier, more vibrant existence.

Appendices

glossary of terms

Blood glucose is the principal sugar contained in the blood and serves as the body's primary source of energy.

The glycemic index (GI) is a measure of how quickly a food raises blood sugar levels.

Glycemic load (GL): a metric that considers both the GI and the carbohydrate content of a serving of food.

Insulin is a hormone generated by the pancreas that regulates blood sugar levels by enabling glucose uptake into cells.

Insulin resistance is a disorder in which the body's cells become less sensitive to insulin, resulting in higher blood sugar levels.

HbA1c is a measure of average blood sugar levels over the previous 2–3 months that is used to diagnose and manage diabetes.

Continuous Glucose Monitor (CGM): a gadget that monitors blood sugar levels all day and night.

Hypoglycemia is defined as low blood sugar levels, which can cause symptoms such as shakiness, perspiration, and confusion.

Hyperglycemia is defined as high blood sugar levels that, if not treated effectively, can lead to long-term health issues.

Endocrine disruptors are chemicals that can interfere with the endocrine (hormonal) system, impacting a variety of biological systems.

Resources and Further Reading

Books:
Dr. Jason Fung's "The Diabetes Code"
"The End of Diabetes" by Dr. Joel Fuhrman .
Dr. Mark Hyman's "The Blood Sugar Solution"

Websites:
American Diabetes Association (www.diabetes.org)
Diabetes UK (www.diabetes.org.uk)
Diabetes can be found at www.cdc.gov/diabetes.

Research journals:
Diabetes Care (American Diabetes Association).
The Journal of Clinical Endocrinology and Metabolism
- Diabetes

Recipe Index.

1. Breakfast:
Greek yogurt with berries and nuts.
Vegetable Omelette and Whole Grain Toast

2. Lunch:
Quinoa salad with mixed greens and grilled chicken.
Lentil soup with spinach and carrots.

3. Dinner:
Baked salmon with roasted vegetables.
Stir-Fried Tofu with Broccoli and Brown Rice

4. Snacks:
Apple slices with almond butter.
Carrot and celery sticks with hummus

Author's Note

Thank you for going on this adventure with me. Writing this book has been a labor of love, motivated by a desire to provide people with the knowledge and tools they need to take charge of their health. I hope this book has given you useful ideas and practical strategies for managing your blood sugar levels properly.

Remember that everyone's journey is unique, so determine what works best for you. Be curious, be driven, and never be afraid to seek help when required. Your health is worth the work, and I am grateful to be a part of your journey.

References

cited studies and articles

1. American Diabetes Association. Diabetes Medical Care Standards for 2021. Diabetes Care, 2021.

2. Centers for Disease Control and Prevention. National Diabetes Statistics Report: 2020.

3. Holt, Richard I. G., et al. Type 1 diabetes management in adults. British Medical Journal, 2021.

4. Miller, V. J. et al., A review of the ketogenic diet's effects on insulin resistance and type 2 diabetes. Journal of Nutrition and Metabolism (2018).

5. Sainsbury, E., et al., The Role of Exercise in Type 2 Diabetes Management: A Review. Diabetes Spectrum: 2018.

Recommended books and articles:

1. "The Diabetes Code," written by Dr. Jason Fung
2. "The End of Diabetes" by Dr. Joel Fuhrman .
3. "The Blood Sugar Solution" by Dr. Mark Hyman
4. "Dr. Bernstein's Diabetes Solution" by Richard K. Bernstein.
5. "Bright Spots & Landmines: The Diabetes Guide I Wish Someone Had Handed Me," written by Adam Brown